Mayo Clinic on
Incontinence

MAYO CLINIC PRESS

Charles County Public Library
P.D. Brown Memorial Library
301-645-2864 301-843-7688
www.ccplonline.org

MAYO CLINIC PRESS

Medical Editors | Paul D. Pettit, M.D., Anita H. Chen, M.D.
Publisher | Daniel J. Harke
Editor in Chief | Nina E. Wiener
Senior Editor | Karen R. Wallevand
Art Director | Stewart J. Koski
Illustration, Photography and Production | Paul W. Honermann, Daniel J. Hubert, Joanna R. King, Michael A. King, Amanda J. Knapp, M. Alice McKiney
Editorial Research Librarians | Abbie Y. Brown, Edward (Eddy) S. Morrow Jr., Erika A. Riggin, Katherine (Katie) J. Warner
Copy Editors | Miranda M. Attlesey, Alison K. Baker, Nancy J. Jacoby, Julie M. Maas
Indexer | Steve Rath
Contributors | Heidi K. Chua, M.D.; Candace F. Granberg, M.D.; Amy E. Krambeck, M.D.; Deborah J. Lightner, M.D.; Cynthia E. Neville, P.T., D.P.T., W.C.S.; John A. Occhino, M.D.; Randina Harvey-Springer, APRN, C.N.P.; Emanuel C. Trabuco, M.D.

Image Credits | The individuals pictured are models, and the photos are used for illustrative purposes only. All photographs and illustrations are copyright of MFMER except for the following: NAME: shutterstock_297786143.eps/PAGE: COVER/CREDIT: © SHUTTERSTOCK NAME: shutterstock_1317987359.eps/PAGE: COVER/CREDIT: © SHUTTERSTOCK NAME: shutterstock_461056675.jpg/PAGE: 24/CREDIT: © SHUTTERSTOCK NAME: shutterstock_631243319.jpg/PAGE: 28/CREDIT: © SHUTTERSTOCK NAME: shutterstock_1532815931.jpg/PAGE: 41/CREDIT: © SHUTTERSTOCK NAME: shutterstock_492832387.jpg/PAGE: 56/CREDIT: © SHUTTERSTOCK NAME: shutterstock_1193218570.jpg/PAGE: 58/CREDIT: © SHUTTERSTOCK NAME: shutterstock_1013316427.jpg/PAGE: 60/CREDIT: © SHUTTERSTOCK NAME: shutterstock_1195916284.jpg/PAGE: 68/CREDIT: © SHUTTERSTOCK NAME: shutterstock_1238330020.jpg/PAGE: 75/CREDIT: © SHUTTERSTOCK NAME: shutterstock_1071960113.jpg/PAGE: 109/CREDIT: © SHUTTERSTOCK NAME: shutterstock_1038733552.jpg/PAGE: 118/CREDIT: © SHUTTERSTOCK NAME: shutterstock_586592117.jpg/PAGE: 119/CREDIT: © SHUTTERSTOCK NAME: shutterstock_1332449717.jpg/PAGE: 123/CREDIT: © SHUTTERSTOCK NAME: shutterstock_52420438.jpg/PAGE: 132/CREDIT: © SHUTTERSTOCK NAME: shutterstock_1125903149.jpg/PAGE: 139/CREDIT: © SHUTTERSTOCK NAME: shutterstock_1402173971.jpg/PAGE: 143/CREDIT: © SHUTTERSTOCK NAME: shutterstock_248168239.jpg/PAGE: 160/CREDIT: © SHUTTERSTOCK NAME: shutterstock_491538292.jpg/PAGE: 171/CREDIT: © SHUTTERSTOCK NAME: shutterstock_428789692.jpg/PAGE: 178/CREDIT: © SHUTTERSTOCK NAME: shutterstock_1080411422.jpg/PAGE: 182/CREDIT: © SHUTTERSTOCK NAME: shutterstock_1683359032.jpg/PAGE: 186/CREDIT: © SHUTTERSTOCK

Published by Mayo Clinic Press

© 2021 Mayo Foundation for Medical Education and Research (MFMER)

MAYO, MAYO CLINIC and the Mayo triple-shield logo are marks of Mayo Foundation for Medical Education and Research. All rights reserved. No part of this book may be reproduced, stored in a retrieval system, or transmitted, in any form or by any means, electronic, mechanical, photocopying, recording or otherwise, without the prior written permission of the publisher.

The information in this book is true and complete to the best of our knowledge. This book is intended only as an informative guide for those wishing to learn more about health issues. It is not intended to replace, countermand or conflict with advice given to you by your own physician. The ultimate decision concerning your care should be made between you and your doctor. Information in this book is offered with no guarantees. The author and publisher disclaim all liability in connection with the use of this book.

For bulk sales to employers, member groups and health-related companies, contact Mayo Clinic, 200 First St. SW, Rochester, MN 55905 or email SpecialSalesMayoBooks@mayo.edu.

ISBN 978-1-893005-71-6

Library of Congress Control Number: 2020952435

Printed in the United States of America

Some images within this content were created prior to the COVID-19 pandemic and may not demonstrate proper pandemic protocols. Please follow all recommended CDC guidelines for masking and social distancing.

Table of Contents

Preface

This book is intended to be a source of hope and assurance for all individuals who experience bladder and bowel control problems. Our message is that incontinence isn't something that you need to live with. Most incontinence can be improved or cured.

No matter how bothersome your symptoms — whether your incontinence is more of an annoyance or it's severe enough that you're afraid to leave the house — there are steps that you can take to manage or treat the problem. Incontinence shouldn't keep you from enjoying an active life.

A variety of therapies — from lifestyle changes to minimally invasive procedures to surgery — can help with bladder and bowel problems.

A number of advances have been made in the treatment of both urinary and fecal incontinence. Newer medications have been approved, and additional nonprescription products are now available. Minimally invasive treatments such as bulking agents and Botox injections provide added treatment options. Procedures such as sacral nerve stimulation are seeing greater use. In addition, advances have been made in surgical procedures to treat more-severe symptoms.

We hope this book helps you gain a better understanding of incontinence and that it serves as a guide to effective medical care so that you can lead a full and active life.

Paul D. Pettit, M.D.
Anita H. Chen, M.D.
Medical Editors

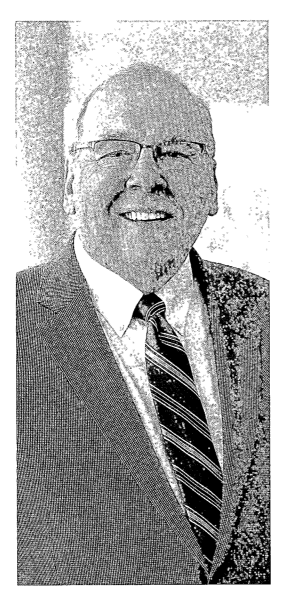

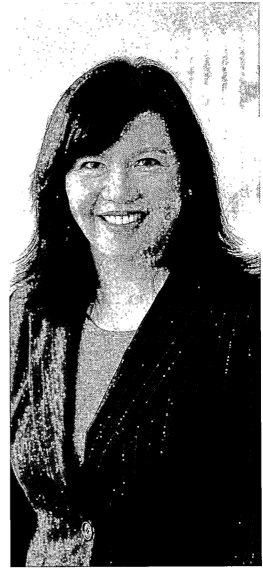

Paul D. Pettit, M.D., has been a gynecologic surgeon at Mayo Clinic in Jacksonville, Fla., for 35 years. Dr. Pettit is board-certified in female pelvic medicine and reconstructive surgery. He initiated development of the Gynecologic Continence Program at Mayo Clinic in Jacksonville.

Anita H. Chen, M.D., is a urogynecologist at Mayo Clinic in Jacksonville, Fla. Dr. Chen is board-certified in obstetrics and gynecology and female pelvic medicine and reconstructive surgery.

Getting help

For many people, taking that initial step to treat incontinence is the most difficult part. Where do you go? Who do you see? If you have a primary care provider, making an appointment with him or her is probably a good place to start. Family practitioners, general internists, physician assistants and nurse practitioners often can treat incontinence, especially mild symptoms.

However, not all primary care providers have the interest, training or experience to treat the condition. And some may take the view that incontinence is an inevitable consequence of aging.

If your primary care doctor doesn't seem to have a positive attitude about treating your condition, he or she seems uninformed when discussing the subject, or

you just don't feel satisfied that you're receiving appropriate care, you might find it most helpful to see a specialist.

Who specializes in treatment for incontinence? There are a few different options. The specialist you should see depends on the type of incontinence you have and whether you're male or female.

- **Female pelvic medicine and reconstructive surgery specialist.** This is a newer medical subspecialty. An individual with these credentials is an obstetrician-gynecologist (OB-GYN) or a urologist with additional training in diseases and disorders affecting the female pelvic floor. The pelvic floor is the network of muscles, ligaments, tissue and nerves that help support and control the rectum, uterus, vagina and bladder. A female pelvic medicine and reconstructive surgery specialist — previously known as a urogynecologist — has passed board examinations in this specialty area and is certified to treat women with complex benign pelvic conditions, lower urinary tract disorders, pelvic floor dysfunction and defecation disorders. You might ask to be referred to such a specialist if an individual with this type of training is available within your care network.

- *Obstetrician-gynecologist.* Obstetrician-gynecologists (OB-GYNs) are trained in caring for women. Many can manage or treat simple types of urinary leakage. If there isn't a female pelvic medicine and reconstructive surgery specialist at your clinic or hospital, you may want to see an OB-GYN.
- *Urologist.* A urologist specializes in male reproductive organs and urinary disorders in both men and women. Men with urinary incontinence generally are treated by a urologist.
- *Gastroenterologist.* A gastroenterologist is trained to treat conditions of the digestive (gastrointestinal or GI) tract in both men and women — including fecal incontinence. You may see a specialist known as a motility specialist within the gastroenterology department. This individual has expertise in conditions that interfere with the coordinated contractions that move food and waste through the digestive tract.
- *Colorectal surgeon.* For some fecal disorders, you may be referred to a colorectal surgeon. If you have a defecation disorder that's resulting from a problem with the pelvic floor muscles, you may need to be treated by a surgeon.

HOW TO USE THIS BOOK

The purpose of this book is to allow you to discuss incontinence and its treatment options with your provider in a more informed manner, so that together you can make the best choices for your care.

Part 1

Part 1 focuses on urinary incontinence. In this section, you'll learn about the many causes of urinary incontinence, the different types of urinary incontinence and the tests used to help diagnose the cause of your symptoms. Most importantly, you'll learn about a variety of options for treating urinary incontinence, from conservative approaches to surgery.

Part 2

Part 2 is devoted to fecal incontinence. Similar to Part 1, this section discusses causes of fecal incontinence and the tests used to diagnose it. The last chapter outlines treatment options ranging from behavioral therapies to surgery.

Appendix

The appendix is a quick-reference section that offers tips and advice you may be able to use on a more regular basis. Included in the appendix are sample diaries, lists of foods and medications that may aggravate your condition, and instructions on how to perform specific drills and exercises.

Urinary incontinence

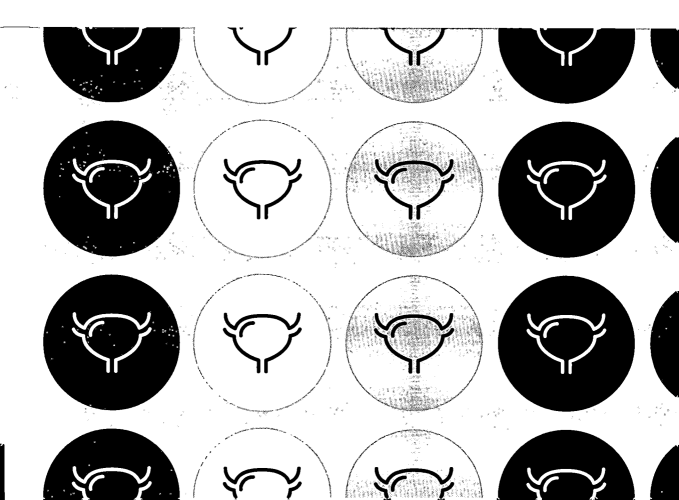

PART 1

Understanding urinary incontinence

1

Here's the truth. Despite what you may think or have been told, loss of bladder control (urinary incontinence) isn't a normal part of childbearing or aging. It has many causes, some of them relatively simple and temporary and others more involved and long-term. And although it's a medical condition, urinary incontinence can also affect other aspects of your life, including your finances and psychological well-being.

The good news is, urinary incontinence can be treated, and in some cases, even cured. And even if treatment can't eliminate the cause of the condition, proper action can ease the discomfort and inconvenience of incontinence and improve your quality of life. With today's medical advances, most people with urinary incontinence can be helped.

Americans spend billions of dollars each year to treat and control urinary incontinence. Most of this money goes toward absorbent pads and other products for managing the condition. The remainder is spent on doctor visits and treatment. If you're living with urinary incontinence, you may know all too well how the condition can affect your pocketbook.

Loss of bladder control can also take an emotional toll. Embarrassment associated with the condition can lead to social withdrawal, depression, anxiety and even sexual dysfunction. Studies indicate that women with severe urinary incontinence are likely to experience depression, and the risk of anxiety is greater among all individuals with loss of bladder control — both women and men — compared with individuals who aren't incontinent.

If you have bladder control problems, you may be reluctant to talk with your doctor about it. Many people experiencing urinary incontinence don't report the problem to their doctors or other medical professionals.

You may be embarrassed to talk about it, as many people are. Or maybe you've convinced yourself that your bladder problem is something you just have to live with. You may believe the common misconception that urinary incontinence is an inevitable consequence of childbearing, menopause, prostate disease or just growing older — and that it's a waste of time to try to do anything about it. Even some doctors take this view.

Don't let embarrassment get the better of you. See your doctor or other medical provider. If he or she doesn't have a positive attitude about treating your condition, seek another medical professional, perhaps someone who specializes in treating incontinence (see page 8).

Although urinary incontinence isn't a disease, it often indicates an underlying condition that often can be treated. A thorough evaluation by a specialist can help determine what's behind your incontinence. Once you've taken that important first step, you'll be well on your way to regaining your confidence and living a more active life.

A COMMON PROBLEM

Urinary incontinence — the inability to control the release of urine from the blad-der — is common. Millions of Americans are affected by the condition. According to the most recent figures from the Centers for Disease Control and Prevention, a significant percentage of adults age 65 and older living independently report some degree of bladder leakage. The problem affects both women and men but is more common in women. More than half of women age 65 and older living independently deal with urinary leakage on a regular basis.

There are a number of reasons why women are more likely to experience loss of bladder control. First of all, the urethra — the tube that runs from the bladder to the urethral opening — in women is much shorter than in men (see the illustration on the opposite page). That means women's urine has a shorter distance to travel to cause leakage. In addition, pregnancy and childbirth can weaken or damage the muscles in the lower pelvis that support the uterus, bladder and bowel, known as the pelvic floor muscles. Pregnancy and childbirth can also weaken the ring of muscles that surrounds the urethra (urethral sphincter). When the muscles weaken, urine may escape whenever pressure is placed on the bladder.

Another reason for the difference is menopause. A reduction in the hormone estrogen that follows menopause affects the organs and tissues of the lower urinary tract. Reduced estrogen can contribute to changes in the linings of the bladder and the urethra, making them less elastic and less able to stay closed. After menopause, the urethral sphincter simply may not be able to hold in urine as easily as it once did, leading to urinary incontinence.

In men, incontinence is more closely associated with aging and age-related health issues. Prostate disease is a significant factor. An enlarged prostate gland (benign prostatic hyperplasia) and treatment for prostate cancer, including prostate surgery, can cause varying degrees of male urinary incontinence.

While urinary incontinence isn't a normal part of aging — that is, it doesn't naturally occur in all individuals as they get older — incontinence is more common with age. Why is this? As you get older, the muscles in your bladder and urethra can lose some of their strength. These age-related changes may reduce the amount of urine your bladder can hold,

which means that you have to urinate more often. And if you don't heed the bathroom call promptly enough, leakage of urine can result.

With age, your pelvic floor muscles also can become weaker, further compromising your ability to hold urine. Some research suggests that your bladder muscle (detrusor) can become overactive as you get older. An overactive bladder muscle creates the urge to urinate before your bladder is full, which can lead to incontinence.

The bottom line: Millions of people experience urinary incontinence every day. Men and women of all backgrounds are affected, some more than others. The good news is that incontinence is treatable — and sometimes curable — for both men and women.

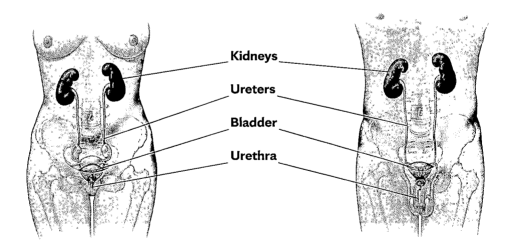

Kidneys

Ureters

Bladder

Urethra

The female (left) and male (right) urinary tracts are essentially the same. The main difference is that in women the urethra is shorter than it is in men.

YOUR URINARY SYSTEM

To understand urinary incontinence, it helps to have some basic knowledge about how the organs and other structures that make up the urinary system work.

When you eat and drink, your body breaks down what you consume into substances that are absorbed into your bloodstream. As your blood circulates, your body's cells absorb liquid and nutrients from your blood and deposit excess fluid and waste in your blood-stream.

The job of your urinary system is to remove, collect, store and eliminate this excess fluid and waste from your blood — and, ultimately, your body — through the process of urination.

Upper urinary system

Your urinary system has two main parts — upper and lower. The upper urinary system consists of two kidneys, each attached to a long, muscular tube called a ureter.

The kidneys are your body's primary filtration system, removing excess fluid and waste from your bloodstream to make urine. Adult-size kidneys filter about 50 gallons of blood each day and make about 2 quarts of urine. The ureters carry the urine to the bladder, delivering it continuously in small, steady amounts. Gravity and the contraction of muscles in the ureter walls force the urine through the long tubes to the bladder.

Lower urinary system

Your lower urinary tract consists of the bladder, a slender drainage tube at the bladder's base called the urethra, and two ring-like bands of muscles at the junction of the bladder and urethra called the internal and external urethral sphincters.

The bladder — a muscular, balloonlike sac — stores urine. When you urinate, the bladder muscle contracts, pushing urine out and through the urethra.

In women, the urethra is about 1½ inches long and it opens to the outside of the body just above the vaginal opening. In men, the urethra is about 8 inches long. The male urethra passes through the walnut-shaped prostate gland at the base of the bladder and through the entire

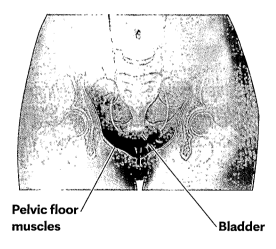

Pelvic floor muscles   **Bladder**

The pelvic floor muscles stretch across the pelvis and support structures of the lower abdomen, including the bladder. When pelvic floor muscles become weakened, urinary incontinence may result.

length of the penis before ending at the tip of the penis.

The urethral sphincters help control the release of urine. The internal sphincter is made up of muscles over which you have no control, called involuntary muscles. It keeps your urethra closed while your bladder is filling, preventing urine from leaking out. This happens with no conscious effort on your part.

When your bladder is nearly full, the internal sphincter automatically relaxes, responding to a message from the brain's bladder control center. That's when the external sphincter goes to work. Made up of muscles that you can consciously control (voluntary muscles), the external sphincter counters the relaxing action of the internal sphincter, helping you keep the urethra closed until you can get to the bathroom to urinate.

Playing a supporting role in all of this are the pelvic floor muscles. They form a hammock-like network of muscles that extends from your pubic bone in the front of your pelvis to your tailbone at the base of your spine. The pelvic floor muscles also extend sideways and attach to the inside of your pelvic bones.

When you urinate, the pelvic floor muscles relax, allowing urine to pass out of your body easily. When you're not urinating, the pelvic floor muscles lightly contract, holding in urine and supporting

BLADDER RELAXED   **BLADDER CONTRACTED**

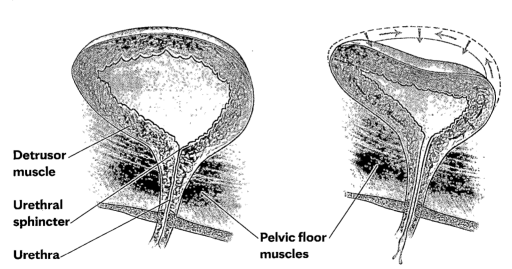

Detrusor muscle

Urethral sphincter

Urethra

Pelvic floor muscles

The detrusor muscle surrounds the bladder. When it contracts (right), and when the urethral sphincter at the base of the bladder relaxes, urine flows through the urethra.

your bladder from underneath. Nerves that run from the spinal cord to the bladder coordinate the action of the pelvic floor muscles. Because these muscles are under voluntary control, they can be strengthened with exercise (see "Pelvic floor exercises" on page 179).

Normal urination

Normal urination is a coordinated process involving the many organs, tubes, muscles and nerves in your urinary system. Once the bladder is nearly full, nerves located in the bladder wall send a signal to the brain. The brain responds with a message to relax the internal urethral sphincter. This creates an urge to urinate. Upon feeling the urge, you decide if it's the appropriate time and place to go to the bathroom.

When you decide to urinate, several things happen. The internal urethral sphincter, the pelvic floor muscles and the external urethral sphincter all relax. At the same time, the bladder contracts, causing pressure inside the bladder to increase. This pushes urine into the urethra. As the bladder wall muscle contracts, urine passes through the urethra and out of your body.

Having good bladder control isn't as simple as it may seem. Urination is a complex process that involves relaxing some muscles while contracting others. The muscles, nerves, organs and tubes in your urinary system must work together. If any part malfunctions, incontinence can result.

TYPES OF URINARY INCONTINENCE

Urinary incontinence is classified by your symptoms or the circumstances at the time you leak urine. The five main types are stress incontinence, urge incontinence, mixed incontinence, overflow incontinence and functional incontinence.

Stress incontinence

Stress incontinence refers to leakage of urine that results when you exert pressure, or stress, on your bladder by coughing, sneezing, laughing, exercising, changing positions or lifting something heavy. It has nothing to do with psychological stress.

Leakage from stress incontinence occurs even though your bladder muscles aren't contracting, and you may not feel the urge to urinate. The problem is especially noticeable when your bladder becomes too full. Actions such as coughing, laughing or exerting yourself may cause a little urine to squirt out or may cause an even larger release.

Physical findings can help doctors determine the subtype of stress incontinence you may have. There are two main subtypes — urethral hypermobility and intrinsic sphincteric deficiency.

Urethral hypermobility

This condition results when the bladder and the urethra shift downward in response to increased abdominal pressure and there isn't enough support from the hammock-like pelvic floor muscles to help keep the urethra closed. As a result, urine leaks out when you cough, sneeze or laugh.

Intrinsic sphincteric deficiency

With this subtype of stress incontinence, there's a problem with your sphincter that keeps it from closing completely or that allows it to open under pressure, leaving your urethra open like a drainpipe. This, too, causes urine to leak out when you cough, sneeze, laugh or otherwise increase the pressure in your abdomen.

In women, stress incontinence may result when the pelvic floor muscles and nerves are weakened or damaged during pregnancy and childbirth. Some experts believe that women who deliver their children vaginally are at the highest risk of developing stress incontinence, although not all studies support this view. Aging and decreased estrogen associated with menopause also are known to contribute to the condition.

In men, the most common cause of stress incontinence is damage to the urethral sphincter, which can occur during surgery, such as surgery for prostate cancer.

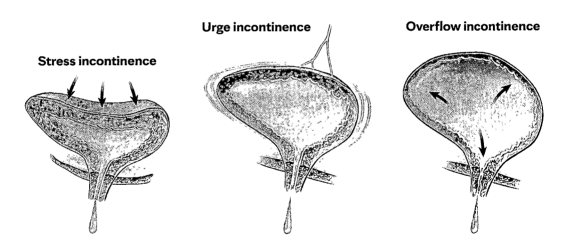

Stress incontinence   **Urge incontinence**   **Overflow incontinence**

With stress incontinence (left), urine leaks when you exert pressure on the bladder when coughing, sneezing, laughing, lifting or simply getting out of bed. With urge incontinence (center), the bladder muscle contracts too often, signaling your brain that you have to urinate. It's characterized by a sudden, involuntary loss of bladder control. Overflow incontinence (right) is characterized by frequent urination or dribbling of urine.

People with lung conditions that cause frequent coughing, such as emphysema, often develop stress incontinence. Coughing places stress on the urinary sphincter. Longtime smokers may experience stress incontinence for this reason.

Urge incontinence

Urge incontinence — sometimes referred to as an overactive bladder — is often characterized by a sudden, intense urge to urinate, followed by an involuntary loss of urine. When your bladder muscles contract, you may have only a few seconds to a minute to reach a bathroom.

It's also common for individuals with urge incontinence to need to urinate frequently, including several times throughout the night (nocturia). Normally, you urinate five or six times a day, with your bladder holding as much as 2 cups of urine. With urge incontinence, you may urinate more than eight to 10 times a day, all in small amounts.

Symptoms of urge incontinence occur when the bladder muscles contract too often and at inappropriate times — namely, when your bladder isn't full. Your brain gets the message that you have to go — and go right away!

Some individuals experience symptoms of urgency and frequency without leakage of urine, but for most people leakage is common. Some people with urge incontinence leak urine when they hear running water or after they drink only a small amount of liquid. Putting your hands under running water to wash dishes may even cause you to leak urine.

Another common problem is what's called the key-in-the-lock syndrome or garage door syndrome. Because you associate arriving home with being able to go to the bathroom, literally as you put your key in the lock or open the garage door, you may feel an overwhelming urge to urinate that causes you to leak urine.

Urge incontinence may result from a urinary tract infection or from something that irritates the bladder. It can also stem from bowel problems or damage to the nervous system associated with a variety of diseases or conditions, such as multiple sclerosis, diabetes, Parkinson's disease, Alzheimer's disease, stroke, or a brain, spine or nerve injury.

In women, urge incontinence typically occurs after menopause, perhaps as a result of bladder changes associated with decreased estrogen levels. In men, urge incontinence may result from a prostate infection or an enlarged prostate gland (benign prostatic hyperplasia). It's also associated with procedures to treat prostate cancer, including freezing the prostate gland (cryotherapy) or radiation-seed treatment (brachytherapy). Often, the cause isn't known — bladder muscles contract (spasm) involuntarily for unknown reasons.

Mixed incontinence

Mixed incontinence means having more than one type of incontinence, typically stress incontinence and urge incontinence. You experience signs and symptoms of both types. You may leak urine when you cough, sneeze or laugh — an activity in which the pressure in your abdomen overcomes what the bladder and urethra can hold back — signaling stress incontinence. And you may also have accidents in which you have a strong urge to urinate and can't reach the toilet in time — signaling urge incontinence.

With mixed incontinence, one type is typically more bothersome than is the other, and the cause of the two forms may or may not be related.

The combination of stress incontinence and urge incontinence most often occurs in women. In fact, some experts suggest that the majority of women with urinary incontinence have signs and symptoms of both stress and urge incontinence. But mixed incontinence isn't an exclusive problem to women. Men who've had their prostate glands removed or who've had surgery for an enlarged prostate can develop mixed incontinence. Older adults also often experience a combination of stress and urge incontinence.

Overflow incontinence

With overflow incontinence, you frequently or even constantly dribble small amounts of urine throughout the day. And when going to the bathroom, you may feel that you need to urinate more — that your bladder isn't empty — but you aren't able to release any more urine. In addition, when you try to urinate, you may have trouble getting started and may produce only a weak stream of urine. Leakage of urine may or may not be accompanied by an urge to go to the bathroom.

Overflow incontinence stems from the inability to completely empty your bladder. Over time, urine accumulates until it exceeds your bladder's capacity to hold it. The increased pressure at the base of your bladder becomes too much to bear. The pressure forces your urethral sphincter to open, and urine leaks out.

Incomplete bladder emptying can occur if your urethra is blocked in some way, obstructing the normal flow of urine from your bladder. Overflow incontinence may also be the result of weak bladder muscles that don't contract forcefully or often enough to empty the bladder and maintain normal urination. Think of this as the opposite of urge incontinence caused by an overactive bladder.

Overflow incontinence is common among men with prostate gland problems. The prostate gland, which surrounds the urethra, commonly enlarges. As it does, it may narrow or block the urethra, preventing the bladder from emptying. Tumors, bladder stones and scar tissue also can block the urethra, keeping urine from leaving the bladder normally.

Nerve damage from diabetes, multiple sclerosis, shingles, injury or other diseases can lead to overflow incontinence. Damaged nerves can cause weak bladder muscles, which don't contract normally during urination. Medications that prevent your bladder from contracting normally or that make you unaware of the urge to urinate also can cause or increase overflow incontinence. These may include painkillers, antidepressants and smooth muscle relaxants. (For a list of medications that may cause or worsen urinary incontinence, see page 178.)

Overflow incontinence is fairly rare among women. It can occur as the result of nerve damage sustained during childbirth, from radical pelvic surgery for cancer, or from certain medical conditions such as diabetes. In addition, women with severe uterine or bladder prolapse may experience overflow incontinence. With the uterus or bladder sagging out of its proper position (see page 95), the urethra can become kinked, interfering with urine flow.

If left untreated, overflow incontinence can have serious consequences. The urine that's retained in the bladder can become infected, and this infection may spread throughout the entire urinary system. In severe cases, urine can back up into the kidneys, damaging the kidneys and affecting kidney function.

Functional incontinence

Functional incontinence is the inability to make it to the bathroom in time because of a physical impairment, mental illness or a disability that's unrelated to your urinary system. For example, if you have severe arthritis in your hands, you may not be able to unbutton your pants quickly enough, and you may leak urine. If you're in a wheelchair or you have trouble walking, getting to a toilet quickly may be difficult. Even though your urinary system is functioning properly, you may frequently have accidents in which you wet your pants.

Many of the conditions that lead to functional incontinence are associated with aging. Dementia, including Alzheimer's disease, can affect urination by causing difficulty in finding a toilet or confusion about how to use it.

Your home environment also may be a problem. Having a bathroom that's too far away — especially if it's upstairs and there are no handrails — can be a hindrance in getting to the bathroom in time. Sometimes, just the fear of falling is enough to prevent an older person from going upstairs to use the toilet.

Medications can sometimes lead to functional incontinence. Diuretics used to treat high blood pressure or congestive heart failure can cause you to produce abnormally large amounts of urine. Some medications can also decrease your awareness of the need to find a toilet.

Functional incontinence that's triggered by medications is sometimes referred to as transient incontinence because changing or discontinuing the medication may solve the problem.

Not surprisingly, many older adults in nursing homes are incontinent, and functional incontinence is a common cause.

Urinary incontinence is described in a variety of ways. Other types of urinary incontinence include:

- **Reflex incontinence.** This form of incontinence occurs among people with serious neurological impairment, such as those with the birth defect spina bifida or with paralysis from a spinal cord injury that affects the nerves running to the bladder. Damage to these nerves prevents the transfer of messages between the brain and the bladder, leading to urine loss without any sensation or warning.
- **Total incontinence.** Total incontinence is another term used to describe continuous leaking of urine day and night, or periodic leakage of large volumes of urine. People with this type of incontinence may have been born with a physical defect or experienced a spinal cord injury or injury to the urinary system during surgery.
- **Reversible incontinence.** This term may be used to describe urine leakage that's temporary — that should go away when the condition causing it improves. Reversible incontinence has many possible triggers, including a urinary tract infection, medications, temporary mental impairment and severe constipation causing stool impaction.
- **Nocturnal enuresis.** This is the medical term for nighttime bed-wetting. Some children, mainly boys, who are otherwise toilet trained wet the bed at night for a variety of reasons. For more information on childhood bed-wetting, see page 103. Adults can lose control of their bladders at night, as well, possibly because of alcohol or medications. The aging bladder also is more likely to have difficulty storing urine at night. This, coupled with the fact that the kidneys more readily can filter and eliminate fluid when you're lying down, can lead to greater urine production during sleep.

REASONS TO HOPE

It's important not to let the embarrassment and social stigma associated with urinary incontinence keep you from getting help.

Remember, this is a medical condition that in many cases can be successfully treated. In the chapters that follow, you'll learn more about the various types of urinary incontinence, as well as a variety of options for treating incontinence.

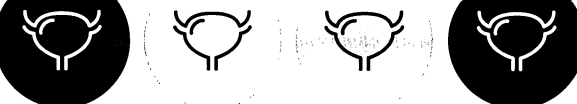
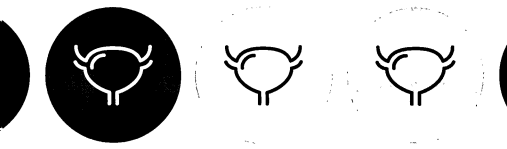
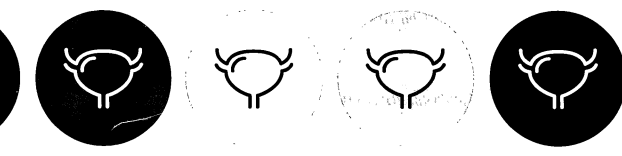
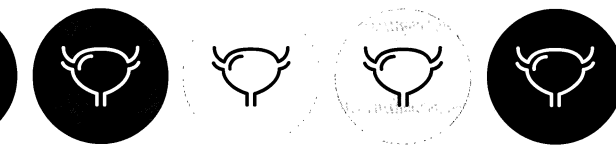
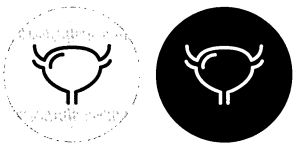
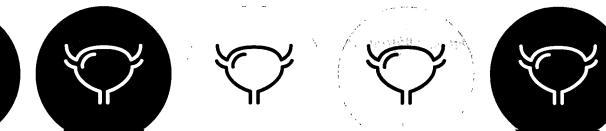

Causes of incontinence

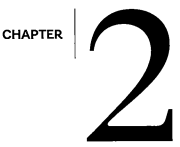

There are many reasons why you may experience bladder control problems. Sometimes the cause may be a temporary problem. In other cases, the problem is a persistent illness or disorder. Persistent causes include underlying physical problems that can't be changed. Temporary (transient) causes can often be reversed with treatment or simple lifestyle changes.

For example, if your incontinence is generally due to the fact that you drink a lot of water and other beverages and then wait until the last minute to go to the bathroom, those are factors that can quite easily be changed. Your incontinence is a temporary problem. Persistent causes of incontinence often include weakened muscles, nerve problems and a variety of medical conditions. The root

problem of these conditions generally can't be reversed. However, that doesn't mean the incontinence can't be treated.

TEMPORARY CAUSES

There are a number of factors that can produce temporary incontinence. Certain foods, beverages or medications can result in incontinence. Temporary incontinence may also be related to an infection or another medical condition that's easily treatable.

Too much fluid

A basic, common cause of incontinence is drinking a lot of fluids, especially in a short period of time. Excessive consumption of

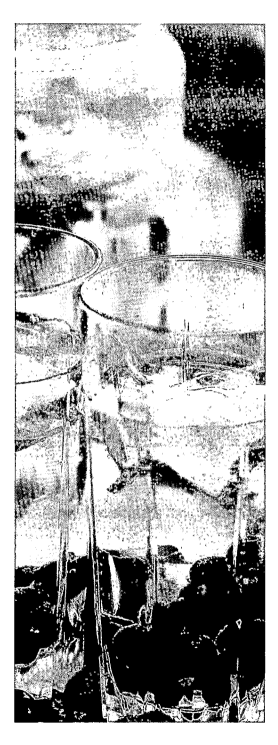

fluids increases the amount of urine your bladder has to retain and release. Polyuria is the medical term for excessive production and output of urine. In addition to drinking large amounts of fluids, consuming caffeinated beverages or alcohol can cause you to urinate a lot. So can certain medications.

If you're producing large amounts of urine, you may not be able to get to the bathroom quickly enough to prevent a wetting accident. If you have to get up several times a night to urinate — and you sometimes don't make it — having to urinate excessively may be to blame.

Treatment involves controlling or correcting the underlying cause of the problem. Reducing how much you drink may help. However, you don't want to cut back on fluids too much. If you don't drink enough fluid, your urine can become concentrated and irritate your bladder. That's not good either.

It's generally recommended that most adults consume approximately 60 ounces of fluid each day. Eight 8-ounce glasses equals 64 ounces. That's easy to remember and a close-enough goal. For some people, fewer than eight glasses might be adequate, and don't forget that you also get fluids from some foods, such as fruits and vegetables.

Alcohol and caffeine

Alcohol and caffeine are diuretics and stimulants. They cause your bladder to produce more urine. As a result, your bladder fills up more quickly than usual and you may experience an urgent, sometimes uncontrollable, need to urinate. Alcohol and caffeine also can irritate the bladder lining, which can lead to incontinence in people with sensitive bladders.

Irritating foods and beverages

Among some individuals, carbonated drinks, fruit and fruit juices can irritate the bladder and may cause episodes of urinary incontinence. Spicy foods, tomato-based products, and foods and beverages containing artificial sweeteners are other common culprits. See page 176 for a list of foods and beverages that can cause bladder irritability.

Medications

Medications are one of the most common causes of urinary incontinence. Some high blood pressure and heart medications can relax bladder muscles, allowing urine to flow more easily and sometimes leak. Other medications — including diuretics — can trigger or worsen incontinence by causing you to make more urine.

Antidepressants and sedatives may worsen incontinence by decreasing your awareness of the need to go to the bathroom. You don't wake up at night when your bladder is telling you it's full. Some antidepressants and cold medications may also keep your bladder from emptying completely.

For a list of medications that may contribute to urinary incontinence, see page 178.

Being overweight

In general, the more you weigh, the more likely you are to experience urinary incontinence. Obesity is a risk factor for urinary incontinence, especially among women.

Being significantly overweight puts constant, increased pressure on your bladder and its surrounding muscles, structures and nerves, weakening them and allowing urine to leak out when you cough, sneeze or lift something heavy (stress incontinence).

Obesity is also thought to be a factor in urge incontinence, although the relationship is not quite as strong. Experts believe that carrying extra weight may reduce blood flow to your bladder or interfere with important nerve impulses.

For people who are overweight and having bladder control problems, losing just 5% to 10% of their body weight may significantly reduce pressure within the abdomen that results in added stress on the bladder.

Poor physical fitness

People who are physically fit tend to have strong pelvic floor muscles. When you're not as fit as you should be, your pelvic floor muscles may be weakened, which may contribute to urinary incontinence.

Becoming more physically active can decrease your risk of incontinence. Studies suggest that men who are physically active are less likely to experience the need to go to the bathroom at night (nocturia) compared with men who don't exercise.

Physical activity appears to be helpful for women, too. Studies indicate that women who are more physically active are less likely to experience urinary incontinence than those who are less physically active. However, women participating in more strenuous sports may experience increased symptoms of urinary incontinence.

There's some speculation that vigorous physical activity may cause urinary incontinence — not protect against it. High-impact sports, such as running or basketball may cause episodes of incontinence in otherwise healthy people. These vigorous activities can put sudden, strong pressure on your bladder, allowing urine to leak past your urethral sphincter. However, no data links high-impact sports to an increased risk of chronic stress incontinence.

Urinary tract infection

A urinary tract infection is an infection that begins in your urinary system, typically in your urethra or bladder or both. A bladder infection is called cystitis. An infection of the urethra is known as urethritis. Urinary tract infections typically occur when bacteria from outside the body enter the urinary tract

through the urethra and begin to multiply in the bladder. The resulting infection irritates the bladder, causing you to experience strong urges to urinate. These urges can be so strong that you can't get to the bathroom in time, resulting in episodes of urinary incontinence.

Having foreign bacteria in your urine does not mean you have a urinary tract infection. In general, urinary tract infections cause incontinence only when they're accompanied by other urinary signs and symptoms, such as a strong, persistent urge to urinate, foul-smelling urine or a burning sensation when urinating.

Urinary tract infection is a common cause of urinary incontinence and is easily reversible with treatment. If your symptoms are typical and you're generally in good health, antibiotics are often the first line of treatment. Usually, symptoms clear up within a few days of treatment.

Other urinary tract problems

Other disorders less commonly responsible for incontinence include an obstruction or a fistula.

Obstruction

A tumor anywhere along your urinary tract can block the normal flow of urine and cause incontinence, usually overflow incontinence. Urinary stones — hard, stonelike masses that can form in the bladder — also may be to blame for urine leakage, especially if a stone interferes with normal urine flow. An obstruction may also result from scar tissue in the urinary tract. Treatment to remove or fix the obstruction often will treat the incontinence.

Urogenital fistula

On rare occasions, women may develop an abnormal opening (fistula) between part of the urinary tract and the vagina, which can cause continuous leakage of urine. A fistula may occur as a result of complicated labor and delivery, surgery, or radiation treatment. Repairing the fistula will often correct the incontinence problem.

Constipation

Chronic constipation can lead to impacted stool — a large mass of dry, hard stool within your rectum. The rectum is located near the bladder and the two share many of the same nerves. Hard, compacted stool in your rectum can cause these shared nerves to become overactive, increasing bladder muscle contractions and urinary frequency. In addition, compacted stool can sometimes interfere with the emptying of the bladder, which may cause overflow incontinence.

Stool impaction is a relatively common cause of urinary incontinence, especially among older adults who may not be getting enough liquid or fiber in their diets. Improving bowel function with dietary changes or stool softeners reduces constipation and urinary leakage problems.

Psychological problems

In rare cases, psychological problems, especially severe depression, may result in urinary incontinence. This may be especially true after major surgery, being diagnosed with a serious illness or experiencing a major loss. Depression can make an individual lose interest in all aspects of personal hygiene, including staying dry.

It's sometimes hard to know, however, whether severe depression is directly to blame for urinary incontinence. If you're recovering from surgery or being treated for a serious illness, you may be taking medications that contribute to incontinence.

Another rare cause of incontinence is delirium, defined as a severely confused mental state. Delirium may result from certain medications, sleep deprivation, and acute illness, such as an infection or kidney or liver failure. Some people also become delirious in reaction to use of anesthesia.

When you're delirious or confused, for whatever reason, you may temporarily lose bladder control. In this context, urinary incontinence is a symptom of an altered mental state. Once the underlying cause of confusion is identified and treated, the problem of incontinence generally goes away.

PERSISTENT CAUSES

There are number of conditions that can lead to persistent urinary incontinence. If your incontinence is due to one of these causes, you may think that's there's not much you can do. That's not true. Even if the root cause of the problem can't be fixed, steps can be taken to help alleviate your symptoms. Here are some of the more common causes of persistent incontinence. Additional information on some of these conditions can be found in Chapter 7.

Pregnancy and childbirth

Pregnant women commonly experience stress incontinence because of hormonal changes that occur with pregnancy and the increased weight of an enlarging uterus on the bladder. Fortunately, after the baby is born, these problems generally go away.

But pregnancy can also lead to persistent incontinence. The stress of a vaginal delivery during childbirth can weaken the muscles needed for bladder control. Childbirth can also damage bladder nerves and supportive tissue, leading to a dropped (prolapsed) pelvic floor. In this condition, the bladder, uterus, rectum or small intestine gets pushed down from its usual position and presses on vaginal walls, causing persistent incontinence (see page 95). Multiple births, prolonged labor, and an episiotomy or use of forceps during childbirth also can further stretch and weaken pelvic floor and urinary sphincter muscles.

Treatment aimed at the pelvic muscles is often the first step in improving pregnancy-related incontinence.

Aging

Urinary incontinence is not a given as you grow older. However, aging is a risk factor for loss of bladder control. Most studies show that the prevalence of urinary

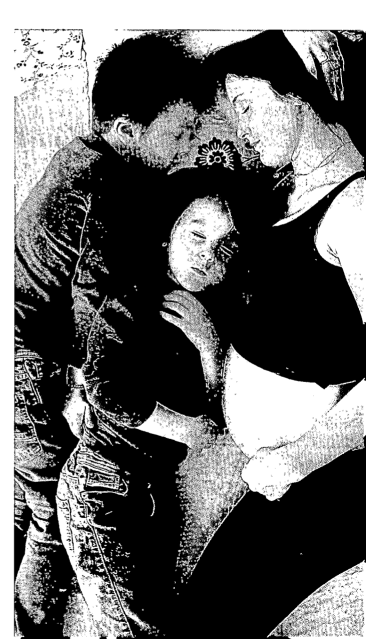

incontinence increases steadily with age. Why is that?

As you get older, many changes occur in the organs, tissues and supporting structures of your urinary system. The muscles in your bladder and urethra lose some of their strength. These age-related changes decrease your bladder's capacity to store urine, which means you have to urinate more often. If you don't heed the call promptly enough, urinary incontinence can result.

Your bladder walls also become less elastic with age — and therefore less able to contract and expel urine. In fact, studies show that compared with younger adults, older adults tend to retain a higher volume of urine in the bladder after urination. This is known as postvoid residual volume, and it can contribute to urinary incontinence. In addition, your pelvic floor muscles may become weaker with age, further compromising your ability to hold urine.

Research also suggests that your bladder muscle (detrusor) becomes more active with age. An overactive bladder muscle creates the urge to urinate before your bladder is full, which can lead to incontinence. In many older adults, the detrusor muscle contracts too often, but the contractions are weak. This condition — called detrusor hyperactivity with impaired contractility — creates the worst of both worlds. You have frequent, sometimes uncontrollable urges to urinate, but you can't quite completely empty your bladder. This can lead to both urge incontinence and overflow incontinence.

As you get older, your kidneys also become less efficient at removing waste from your bloodstream. This decline in filtration can cause you to produce more urine later in the day. In fact, unlike younger people, who produce most of their urine during the day, older adults produce roughly the same amount of urine during the day and at night. Having to urinate several times a night can result in incontinence.

People are also more likely to experience medical conditions as they get older, such as congestive heart failure, diabetes or Alzheimer's disease. All of these conditions can contribute to urinary incontinence. Age-related problems that restrict mobility, such as severe arthritis or a hip fracture, also can lead to the problem.

Menopause

In women, the hormone estrogen helps keep the lining of the bladder and urethra healthy. After menopause, the female body produces less estrogen. The decline in estrogen generally causes the tissues of the urethra and vagina to become drier, thinner, less elastic and more susceptible to irritation. This condition — once known as atrophic urethritis or atrophic vaginitis and now called genitourinary syndrome of menopause — can contribute to urinary incontinence.

Women with the condition typically report increased urinary frequency and urgency, sometimes resulting in urge incontinence. However, the condition can also cause or contribute to stress incontinence. As the tissues of the urethra become thinner, they lose resistance. This can lead to urine leakage when your bladder contains urine and you're upright and active. If you also have weak pelvic floor and sphincter muscles, your risk of urine leakage may be especially high.

The urethral sphincter, in fact, often loses some of its ability to close — meaning it can't hold back urine as easily as it did before. This can cause you to leak urine when you cough, sneeze, laugh, exercise or lift something heavy (stress incontinence). The hormonal changes of menopause can also make women more prone to urinary tract infections, which sometimes can cause urinary incontinence.

Genitourinary syndrome of menopause may be treated with estrogen cream applied to the vaginal area. Vaginal estrogen tablets and rings also are available. The estrogen, which helps to restore vaginal tissue, stays primarily in the vaginal area. Estrogen therapy in pill or patch form is less effective and poses additional risks, especially for women who've had or are at high risk of breast or uterine cancer.

Entering menopause isn't a guarantee that you'll develop bladder problems. Some studies comparing premenopausal and postmenopausal women found no differences in the overall rates of bladder control problems. Research suggests, however, that postmenopausal women tend to have more-frequent problems with urine leakage than do younger women.

Prostate conditions

Among men, incontinence is often related to problems with the prostate gland. For additional information on prostate disease and incontinence, see page 98.

Enlarged prostate

In older men, incontinence often stems from enlargement of the prostate gland, a condition called benign prostatic hyperplasia (BPH). The prostate gland surrounds the urethra. As the gland enlarges, it can constrict the urethra and partially block the flow of urine, weaken-

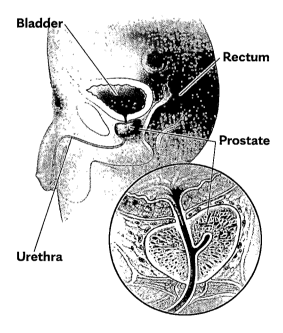

Bladder **Rectum** **Prostate** **Urethra**

The prostate gland surrounds the neck of the bladder and the upper portion of the urethra much like a doughnut.

ing the urine stream and causing a frequent need to urinate. For some men, this problem results in urge or overflow incontinence.

Prostatitis

Loss of bladder control isn't a typical sign of prostatitis, an inflammation of the prostate gland. Even so, urinary incontinence sometimes occurs with this common condition.

Bladder conditions

On occasion, incontinence may result from a bladder disorder.

Bladder cancer

Incontinence may be a sign of bladder cancer, which can produce frequent, sudden urges to urinate. Most often, though, it's other signs and symptoms of bladder cancer that cause an individual to see a doctor. They include blood in the urine, a burning sensation during urination and pelvic pain.

Interstitial cystitis/painful bladder syndrome (IC/PBS)

Interstitial cystitis is a chronic condition characterized by a combination of uncomfortable bladder pressure, bladder pain and pelvic pain. The condition is part of a spectrum of diseases known as painful bladder syndrome.

Pain from interstitial cystitis can range from a mild burning or discomfort to severe pain. The condition, which is most common in women, may also cause a persistent, urgent need to urinate and frequent urination. People with severe IC/PBS may go to the bathroom as often as 60 times a day. Because of the frequent need to urinate, the condition can result in bladder control problems.

Your bladder, you'll recall, is a hollow, muscular organ that stores urine. The bladder expands until it's full and then signals your brain that it's time to urinate, communicating through the pelvic nerves. This creates an urge to urinate for most people. With interstitial cystitis, these signals get mixed up — you feel the need to urinate more often and with smaller volumes of urine in the bladder.

Signs and symptoms of interstitial cystitis vary from person to person. If you have the condition, your symptoms may also vary over time, periodically flaring in response to common triggers, such as menstruation, sitting for a long time, stress, exercise and sexual activity. Some people experience symptom-free periods.

The exact cause of interstitial cystitis isn't known, but it's likely that many factors contribute. For instance, people with interstitial cystitis may also have a defect in the protective lining (epithelium) of the bladder. A leak in the epithelium may allow toxic substances in urine to irritate the bladder wall. Other possible but unproven contributing factors include an autoimmune reaction, heredity, infection or allergy.

There's no cure for IC/PBS, but medications and other therapies may offer relief. The medication pentosan polysulfate sodium (Elmiron) is approved specifically for treating IC/PBS. However, studies are finding that it may lead to eye damage in some individuals. If you take the medication or have in the past, make sure to have your eyes examined.

Surgery

Certain surgeries may increase your risk of incontinence. In women, the bladder and the uterus lie close to each other and are supported by the same muscles and ligaments. In men, the same is true for the bladder and the prostate gland. Not surprisingly, surgery to remove the uterus or prostate gland can lead to incontinence.

Hysterectomy

A possible side effect of surgery involving the female reproductive system — for example, removal of the uterus (hysterectomy) — is damage to the supporting pelvic floor structures, including connective tissue and nerves. This can lead to incontinence.

Having a hysterectomy doesn't mean that you'll develop bladder problems. Studies examining the link between hysterectomy and urinary incontinence have produced conflicting results. Some have found a strong relationship — others have found none at all.

Prostate surgery

Urinary incontinence is a known side effect of prostate surgery. During radical prostatectomy for prostate cancer, a surgeon removes the prostate gland and sometimes the surrounding lymph nodes, while trying to spare the muscles and nerves that control urination and sexual function. On occasion, the urinary sphincter or critical nerves may be damaged.

Most men who've undergone a radical prostatectomy experience bladder control problems. These problems may last for weeks or even months. Some men eventually regain complete bladder control, but others may leak urine when they sneeze, cough, laugh or lift something heavy. Stress incontinence is the most common type of incontinence after radical prostatectomy, but prostate surgery can also sometimes trigger urge incontinence or overflow incontinence. In some men, major urinary leakage persists and additional surgery may be needed to help correct the problem.

Other prostate surgeries also may lead to urinary incontinence. For example, transurethral resection of the prostate (TURP) is the most common surgery to relieve urinary symptoms associated with an enlarged prostate gland. Most men experience a stronger urine flow within a few days after surgery. But in some cases, TURP can cause loss of bladder control. This condition is usually temporary, but it can take up to a year for it to disappear entirely.

For more information on urinary incontinence as it relates to prostate disease, see the section on men's bladder health beginning on page 98.

Other surgeries

Surgery to treat pelvic diseases such as colon, ovarian and cervical cancers also carries a risk of damaging the muscles and nerves of the urinary tract, possibly causing urinary incontinence.

Damage to the nerves supplying the bladder may cause urine retention and overflow incontinence, while damage to the nerves supplying the urethra or the bladder neck may cause stress incontinence.

Radiation treatment

Normally, your bladder stretches as it fills with urine. The fuller it gets, the more it stretches. Radiation therapy to the pelvic area can damage the bladder wall, making it somewhat stiff. This loss of elasticity can cause increased urinary frequency and urgency, and it sometimes results in urinary incontinence.

Radiation damage to the bladder wall can occur after radiation therapy for gynecological, urologic and colorectal cancers. Among men who undergo external beam radiation treatment for prostate cancer, the most common urinary problems are increased urgency and frequency. These problems usually are temporary and gradually diminish within a few weeks of

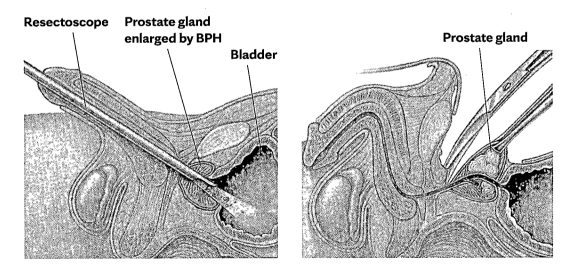

Resectoscope   **Prostate gland enlarged by BPH**   **Bladder**   **Prostate gland**

Incontinence may result from surgery of the prostate gland, including the scraping away of excess tissue within an enlarged prostate to improve urine flow (left) or removal of the gland to treat prostate cancer (right).

completing treatment. Long-term problems are uncommon.

With radioactive seed implants (brachytherapy), it's a slightly different story. Seed implants deliver a higher dose of radiation to the urethra and can cause urinary problems. Some men need medication to treat their symptoms. A few also need intermittent self-catheterization to help them urinate.

In general, severe urinary incontinence isn't a common side effect of seed implants, but some men may experience persistent symptoms.

Restricted mobility

There are many reasons why people have a difficult time getting around. Arthritis, hip pain or foot problems can make it difficult to walk. Other medical problems — such as congestive heart failure, which can make walking exhausting, or poor eyesight — can restrict mobility.

If your ability to get around is restricted to the point you can't respond promptly to the urge to urinate, incontinence can result. In addition, if you have severe arthritis in your hands, you may not have the dexterity necessary to undo fasteners on your clothes in time to avoid urine leakage. In general, the more difficult it is for you to move, the greater your likelihood of experiencing incontinence.

Improving mobility can often improve incontinence. If you have trouble with mobility, talk with your doctor. The underlying problem may be more treatable than you think.

Congestive heart failure

Congestive heart failure often occurs because other cardiovascular diseases have damaged or weakened your heart, forcing it to work harder. The condition can result from a heart attack, high blood pressure or other forms of heart disease, such as valve disorders. Because your heart is weakened, it can't pump blood efficiently. This causes blood to pool in your legs, feet and ankles, causing swelling (edema). Your kidneys also retain excess water and sodium, and fluid backs up into your lungs, leading to shortness of breath.

The accumulation of fluid that occurs with congestive heart failure can also cause or contribute to incontinence. With excess fluid in your body, you have to urinate more frequently. If you're not strong enough to get to the bathroom quickly, an accident can result. Congestive heart failure and edema in your legs and ankles may also lead to increased production of urine at night, which can contribute to urinary incontinence. Sometimes, just the act of lying flat is enough to cause urine leakage. When you lie down, excess fluid moves from your lower extremities, sometimes creating pressure on your bladder and an uncontrollable urge to urinate.

Medications taken to treat congestive heart failure — mainly diuretics — are another potential cause of incontinence.

They prevent fluid from collecting in your body by making you urinate more often.

Diabetes

Diabetes can cause or contribute to urinary incontinence in several different ways. Excess blood sugar (glucose) circulating in your bloodstream draws water from your tissues, making you feel dehydrated. To quench your thirst, you may drink a lot of water and other beverages, leading to more frequent urination and bladder control problems. Uncontrolled diabetes with associated high blood sugar (hyperglycemia) is one of the most common causes of excess urine production.

Diabetes also increases your risk of developing urinary tract infections, which irritate the bladder, causing strong urges to urinate. When the urge is so strong that you can't get to the toilet in time, urinary incontinence can result.

Nerve damage (neuropathy) is another complication of diabetes that can produce urinary incontinence. Damage to the nerves that control urination can cause faulty communication between your brain and your urinary tract. This can result in a reduced sensation to urinate, even when your bladder is full, leading to overflow incontinence.

Nerve damage from diabetes may also prevent your bladder from emptying completely, contributing to overflow incontinence and urinary tract infections. If urinary retention isn't properly treated, urine can back up into your kidneys and possibly cause kidney damage.

Diabetes can also affect your kidneys more generally, damaging the intricate system that filters waste from your blood and eliminates it in your urine. Over time, kidney damage from diabetes (nephropathy) can lead to chronic kidney failure. That, in turn, can cause fluid retention, leading to swollen extremities, congestive heart failure or fluid in your lungs. Urinary incontinence can be another consequence of excess fluid retention.

Neurological disorders

A number of disorders affecting the brain and spinal cord can result in incontinence. They include multiple sclerosis, Parkinson's disease, stroke and Alzheimer's disease. A brain tumor or a spinal injury also can interfere with nerve signals involved in bladder control, causing urinary incontinence.

Disorders of the brain and spinal cord can affect bladder control by interrupting the nerve impulses that normally get sent to the bladder. Neurological disorders may also cause your bladder muscle to become overactive. When the bladder muscle is overactive because of a neurological disease or disorder, the condition is known as neurological hyperreflexia.

Multiple sclerosis

In multiple sclerosis, your immune system mistakenly attacks the myelin sheath surrounding the nerves in your brain and spinal cord. The resulting injury and scarring slows or blocks muscle coordination and other nerve signals, often causing bladder overactivity, urinary frequency and sometimes incontinence. Nerve damage from multiple sclerosis can also make your bladder muscle underactive, contributing to overflow incontinence. The majority of people with multiple sclerosis have urinary problems.

Parkinson's disease

Parkinson's disease occurs when neurons in the area of your brain that controls muscle movement are damaged or destroyed. This can cause both uncontrollable muscle movements (tremors) and muscle stiffness (rigidity).

If you have Parkinson's disease, your bladder muscle may become overactive, contributing to urge incontinence, or it may become underactive, contributing to overflow incontinence. The slowed movement and muscle stiffness associated with Parkinson's disease may also make it difficult to get to the toilet in time.

Stroke

A stroke can contribute to urinary incontinence in several different ways. If the bladder control center of the brain is damaged by the stroke itself or subsequent swelling, you may be unable to sense or suppress the urge to urinate.

Control of your bladder muscle also may be impaired, causing neurological hyperreflexia and urge incontinence.

Depending on its severity, a stroke can also impair your ability to think and speak. These impairments may make you unable to recognize the urge to urinate or communicate that need to a caregiver in a timely way. Urinary incontinence is fairly common after a stroke. However, for many people, the problem improves with time and rehabilitation.

Alzheimer's disease

With Alzheimer's disease, healthy brain tissue degenerates, ultimately causing a loss of memory (dementia) that can be severe enough to interfere with daily functioning. Urinary incontinence tends to become more common as the disease progresses and a person's thinking becomes increasingly impaired.

When people with Alzheimer's disease begin to have bladder control problems, it's generally not because of physical factors. It may be because they've forgotten where the bathroom is located or because they have trouble getting to the bathroom in time. Unlike other neurological disorders, Alzheimer's doesn't appear to cause unstable bladder contractions.

Spinal cord injury

An injury to the spinal cord interferes with your brain's ability to communicate with other parts of your body by way of your nervous system. A spinal cord injury may stem from a sudden, traumatic blow to your spine that fractures, dislocates, crushes or compresses one or more of your vertebrae or from a penetrating wound that cuts your spinal cord.

If you have paralysis from a spinal cord injury that affects the nerves running to the bladder, you may experience reflex incontinence. Damage to these nerves prevents the transfer of messages between the brain and the bladder, leading to urine loss without any sensation or warning.

Spinal stenosis

In spinal stenosis, one or more areas of the spine narrow — especially in the upper or lower back — putting pressure on the spinal cord or on the roots of its branching nerves.

Most often, spinal stenosis results from degenerative changes in the spine related to aging. But tumors, injuries and other diseases also can lead to narrowing in the spinal canal. In severe cases of spinal stenosis, the nerves to the bladder may be affected, leading to partial or complete urinary incontinence. The medical term for this problem is cauda equina syndrome.

Some people experience spine-related problems in their necks. Narrowing in the upper (cervical) spine can cause numbness, weakness or tingling in a leg, foot, arm or hand. In severe cases, nerves to the bladder or bowel may be affected,

leading to incontinence. Cervical spondylosis is the medical term for degenerative changes in the bones (vertebrae) and cartilage of the neck.

Normal pressure hydrocephalus

Normal pressure hydrocephalus is a rare condition characterized by swelling of an area of the brain called the cerebral ventricles. This swelling results from excessive cerebrospinal fluid that accumulates within the skull. The swelling can damage brain tissue, leading to a variety of signs, including dementia, difficulty standing and walking, and urinary incontinence.

Normal pressure hydrocephalus most often occurs in people age 60 years and older. Bladder problems may range from urgency and increased urinary frequency in mild cases to complete loss of bladder control in advanced cases.

THE NEXT STEP

Clearly, urinary incontinence has a variety of causes. But regardless of the underlying cause, there's almost always a treatment that can relieve at least some of the signs and symptoms. In the chapters ahead, you'll read about tests doctors use to diagnose incontinence and treatment options that are available once the cause of your bladder problem is known.

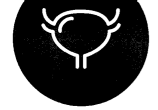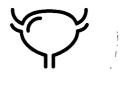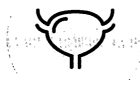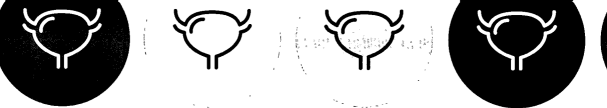

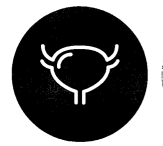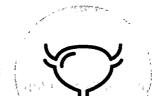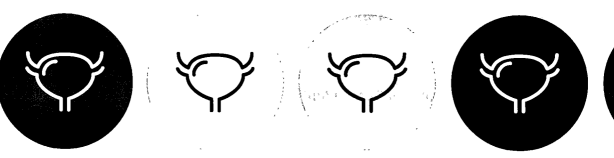

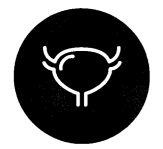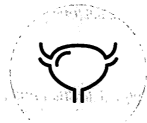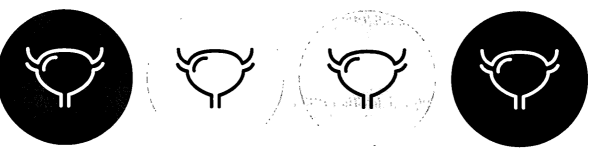

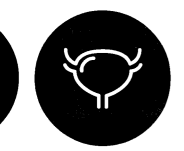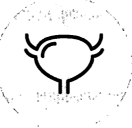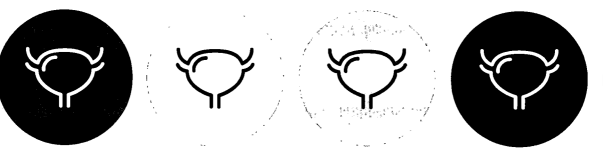

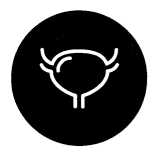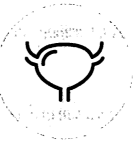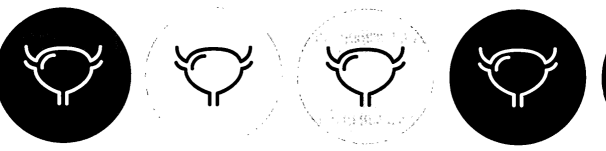

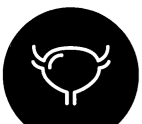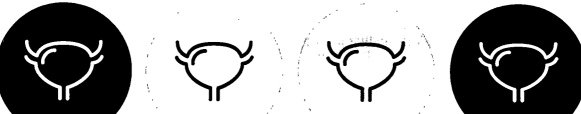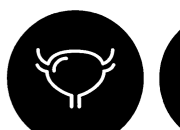

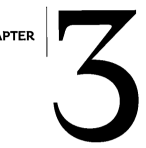

CHAPTER

Evaluation and testing

If you feel uncomfortable discussing urinary incontinence with your doctor or other medical professional, you're not alone — many people do. But seeking medical advice is important for several reasons. First, urinary incontinence may indicate a more serious underlying condition. Second, it may cause you to restrict your activities and keep you from enjoying social events. Third, if you have balance problems, rushing to the bathroom to avoid an accident may put you at risk of falling.

A few isolated accidents don't necessarily require medical attention. But if the problem is frequent or it affects your quality of life, seek help.

On page 8, in the introduction to this book, we discuss the type of doctor you should see to get help for incontinence. If you have a good relationship with your primary care provider, you may want to start with him or her. Otherwise, seek out a specialist.

BEFORE YOUR APPOINTMENT

To get the most from your medical appointment, it helps to be prepared. Good preparation generally consists of two parts. First, document your medical history. This may include getting a copy of your medical record or having it sent to the provider that you'll be seeing. Second, for a week or so, keep a bladder diary — a simple recording of the beverages you consume each day, how much you consume and how often you need to go to the bathroom (see page 174).

This background information will help your medical provider better understand your incontinence so that he or she can more successfully treat it. You may also receive a questionnaire in the mail or electronically about your bladder function. If you do, complete it prior to your appointment and bring it with to the appointment or submit it through your patient portal.

Medical history

Before your visit, review your medical history and make a few lists. Medications are one of the most common causes of urinary incontinence, so list all the medications you're taking. Include prescription drugs, over-the-counter drugs, vitamins, minerals and other supplements. If you're not sure whether something counts as a medication, err on the side of caution and put it on the list.

For each medication, write down both the brand and the generic names, the dose you take, how often you take it, and when you take it. It may also be a good idea to bring your medications with you to your appointment. If you do this, be sure to keep them in their original containers.

In addition, list previous surgeries, births, illnesses, injuries and medical procedures you've undergone, and provide approximate dates. If you have health problems for which you're currently seeing a medical professional or taking medication, such as arthritis or diabetes, list those, too.

For women who've been through menopause, it's also helpful to note when your menstrual periods stopped. If you don't know the date, simply jot down how old you were when you stopped menstruating.

Bladder diary

Before or after your appointment, you may be asked to keep a bladder diary over a several-day period. This is a simple record of "fluids in and fluids out" that may provide important details about your incontinence symptoms.

If you keep it faithfully, the diary will show when you're leaking urine, how often you're leaking, how much you're leaking, how much of an urge is associated with urination and leaking, and which situations in your life seem to be associated with episodes of urinary incontinence.

With the information you record in your diary, your provider may get a better idea of what might be contributing to your incontinence — and how best to treat it. See page 174 for a sample bladder diary.

WHAT TO EXPECT

As with other medical appointments, undergoing a complete medical examination is one of the first steps for urinary incontinence and other bladder symptoms, such as urinary urgency, urinary frequency and waking up at night to urinate (nocturia). The sequence and number of steps in the exam may vary, but it's likely that you'll be asked a series of specific questions about your signs and symptoms, followed by more questions about your medical history.

You'll likely have a complete physical examination and you may undergo some basic tests of your urinary function. The goal is to correlate your signs and symptoms, medical history, physical exam, and test results to provide an accurate assessment of your problem.

Assessing your symptoms

Your appointment will likely begin with a lot of questions about your symptoms. Your answers to these questions can help determine what type of incontinence you have and how best to treat it. If you're unsure about any of your responses, your bladder diary may serve as a helpful resource.

Your provider may first ask about the onset and duration of your symptoms. When did the incontinence start? Did it come on suddenly or more gradually over time? How long has it been going on? Has it gotten any better or worse? Next, there may be questions designed to uncover details about your specific problem.

Here are some questions you may be asked:
- How often do you leak urine during the day? Are you aware that it's happening, or do you just find yourself wet?
- What time of day does it typically occur? Is it worse during the day or at night?

- When you leak urine, is it just a few drops? Or are your clothes or underwear soaked?
- Do you often feel a sudden and intense urge to urinate that's difficult to control?
- Do you feel the urge to urinate when you hear the sound of running water?
- Do you feel the urge to urinate when you put your hands in warm water?
- Do you leak urine when you laugh, cough, sneeze or lift heavy objects?
- Do you leak urine when exercising?
- How often do you urinate each day? Do you urinate more than eight times in a 24-hour period? Do you urinate frequently, but only a small amount each time?
- Do you wake more than once during the night to urinate?

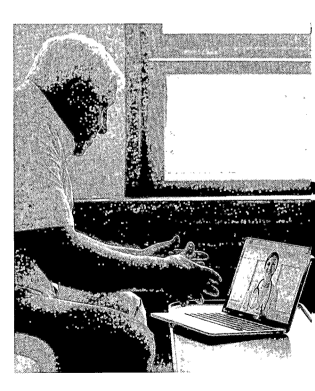

- Do you ever wake up wet?
- Do you feel pain, discomfort, or a burning or smarting sensation while urinating?
- Have you seen blood in your urine?
- Does your urine ever look cloudy?
- Do you have trouble starting the urine stream?
- Do you have a slow or weak urine stream?
- Does your urine stream repeatedly start and stop?
- Does your bladder sometimes feel full even after you urinate?
- Do you have to bear down or strain to urinate?
- Do you dribble urine after you're done urinating?
- How much fluid do you typically drink in a day?
- Do you tend to drink more in the morning, afternoon or evening?
- Do you drink caffeinated beverages? How many each day?
- Do you drink alcoholic beverages? How many each day?
- Have you noticed recent changes in your bowel habits?
- How often do you have bowel movements?
- Are you often constipated?
- Have you had any problems with fecal incontinence?
- Have you noticed any recent changes in your sexual function?
- Do you leak urine during or after sexual intercourse?
- If you're a female, are you still having menstrual periods?
- If you're a female, do you feel vaginal pressure, like your organs have dripped or prolapsed?

- Do you use absorbent pads to protect your clothes from accidents?
- How many pads do you use a day? What type?
- Are the pads usually soaked or just damp?
- Does anything seem to make your incontinence better or worse? If so, what?
- What's the most bothersome aspect of your incontinence?

After your doctor gains a good understanding of your urinary symptoms, the focus turns to what may be causing or contributing to your bladder problems.

The medical history information that you've gathered may help answer many of these questions. Current or past medical problems that can affect bladder control include urinary tract infection, prostate enlargement, diabetes, stroke, Parkinson's disease and multiple sclerosis, among others. For women, menopause also can contribute to urinary incontinence.

You may be asked if you've had surgery or radiation therapy. Gynecological and urologic procedures, such as hysterectomy or radical prostatectomy or radioactive seed implants (brachytherapy) for prostate cancer, are associated with urinary incontinence. It's important to mention all procedures you've had — including any prior surgeries to treat urinary incontinence. Any surgery in which you were catheterized with a Foley catheter may have irritated your urethral lining, which may now be contributing to urinary incontinence.

If you've been pregnant or given birth, you may be asked some questions about that, too. How many times have you been pregnant? How many times have you given birth? What was the size of each baby? Did you deliver vaginally or by cesarean section? Did you have an episiotomy? Were forceps used? Was the birth assisted with a vacuum device? With this information, your doctor will begin to get an idea about the general condition of your pelvic floor muscles.

You may also be asked about medications you're currently taking, including prescriptions, over-the-counter drugs, vitamins, minerals and other supplements. Again, the information you gather to prepare for your appointment should help you answer these questions. Because medications are such a common cause of urinary incontinence, it's important to discuss the subject thoroughly.

After reviewing your specific circumstances, your provider might recommend that some of your medications be reduced, discontinued or taken at different times of the day.

Quality-of-life assessment

Urinary incontinence can cause many unpleasant side effects, such as rashes, skin infections and sores resulting from constantly wet skin. But more distressing may be the effect urinary incontinence can have on your quality of life.

Loss of bladder control may keep you from participating in activities. You may stop exercising, quit attending social gatherings or even refrain from laughing because you're afraid of an accident. You may even reach the point where you stop traveling or you only venture in familiar areas where you know the locations of the bathrooms.

Urinary incontinence can also negatively affect your work life. Constantly going to the bathroom may keep you away from your desk or cause you to have to get up often during meetings. The problem may be so distressing that it disrupts your concentration. Urinary incontinence may also keep you up at night, so you're tired most of the time.

Perhaps most distressing is the effect urinary incontinence can have on your personal life. Your family may not understand the changes in your behavior or may grow frustrated at your many trips to the bathroom. You may avoid sexual intimacy because of embarrassment caused by urine leakage. It's not uncommon for individuals with bladder problems to experience anxiety and depression.

To fully understand how urinary incontinence is affecting your quality of life, your doctor may ask you to complete a questionnaire. The questionnaire asks you to rate how urine leakage has affected different aspects of your life, such as physical recreation, travel, sexual relations and participation in social activities outside your home. In the questionnaire, you may also be asked to describe how leaking urine makes you feel, whether it be nervous, fearful, frustrated, angry, depressed or embarrassed.

Several different questionnaires — sometimes called quality-of-life assessments — are used. These questionnaires serve as tools to help assess the severity of your symptoms, make treatment decisions and get a clearer picture of how your incontinence is affecting your everyday life. This information can help your provider devise treatment strategies to address areas that are most troublesome to you.

PHYSICAL EXAMINATION

A complete physical examination, with extra focus on your abdomen, genital area, rectum and nervous system, can provide important clues to the cause of your incontinence.

Your provider will likely check your vital signs and check for swelling (edema) in your legs, ankles and feet. Lower extremity edema, often a consequence of congestive heart failure, diabetes or kidney failure, contributes to increased urine production at night, which sometimes leads to urinary incontinence.

He or she may also perform a brief neurological exam, testing your reflexes with a reflex hammer and assessing the strength of your leg muscles. You may be asked whether you can feel it when your legs are being touched with a pin — and whether you can distinguish a sharp pin from a duller instrument.

This part of the exam is to try to determine whether neurological disorders such as multiple sclerosis, Parkinson's disease or spinal stenosis may be interrupting or weakening the nerve impulses that normally get sent to your bladder — and therefore contributing to your incontinence.

Your general mobility and dexterity also may be evaluated by observing how easily you can climb onto the examination table or if you have trouble moving about or undressing. These factors could also be contributing to your incontinence.

Stress test

While your bladder is full, a test for stress incontinence may be performed. The test differs slightly between men and women.

Men are asked to stand up and cough. If urine leaks out onto a paper towel, the test is positive for stress incontinence.

Women are asked to cough while lying on the exam table. If no urine leaks out, they're asked to stand up and cough again, bounce on their heels, walk or bend over. You shouldn't be embarrassed if you leak urine during a stress test. Think of it as an important part of beginning to understand your problem.

Once this test is over, you can go to the bathroom so that you're comfortable for the rest of the exam. Be aware that you may be observed you as you urinate to see whether your urine flow is strong and continuous. Sometimes a device may be used to obtain these measurements. If your urine flow is weak and intermittent or if you're straining to urinate, you may have overflow incontinence.

Abdominal exam

Once your bladder is empty, an abdominal exam may follow. If your bladder seems to be larger than it should be (bladder distention), it may mean that it's not emptying completely when you urinate, which could be contributing to overflow incontinence. Soreness or tenderness in the area over your bladder is another symptom of bladder distention. If your provider doesn't hear bowel sounds, you may be constipated, which could be contributing to your incontinence.

An abdominal exam also provides an opportunity to check for other abdominal factors that may be contributing to incontinence, such as a hernia, a tumor, an infection or scarring from previous surgery.

Female exam

In women, a physical exam also focuses on the reproductive organs and rectum. For the exams that follow, you lie on your back on an examining table with your knees bent. Usually, your heels rest in metal supports called stirrups.

Genital exam

Your external genitalia (vulva) and the area between your vulva and anus (perineum) is examined. Chronic exposure to urine can cause skin problems on your perineum and external genitals, such as rashes, sores and infection.

To test the nerves in your genital area, your provider may lightly stroke the perineal skin near your anus and watch or feel for an anal contraction. This reflex is sometimes known as the anal wink. Similarly, lightly tapping on the clitoris can cause an anal contraction. This reflex is known as the bulbocavernosus reflex. If these reflexes aren't normal, it may mean that the nerves in your genital area are somehow contributing to your problem with urinary incontinence. These tests may feel a bit unusual, but they shouldn't be painful.

Internal exam

An internal examination is done to evaluate the condition of your vagina, assess the strength of your pelvic floor muscles, determine whether your bladder or uterus has dropped out of its normal position (pelvic organ prolapse), and detect any abnormal masses. Thinning of vaginal walls (genitourinary syndrome of menopause, or vaginal atrophy), weak pelvic floor muscles, pelvic organ prolapse and abnormal pelvic masses can contribute to urinary incontinence. If prolapse is present, your provider may take measurements to assess its degree.

To begin the internal exam, an instrument called a speculum is inserted into your vagina. With the speculum in the open position, your provider checks for inflammation or discharge, which may suggest a vaginal infection. He or she may also be able to see whether your vaginal walls are thinning. Often, if your vaginal walls are thinning, the tissues lining your urethra are thinning, too, which may contribute to urinary incontinence.

After examining your vagina, your provider may insert one or two gloved fingers into your vagina to help assess the strength of your pelvic floor muscles and determine if your bladder and uterus are in the proper position. Some providers use a speculum to do this portion of the exam. You may be asked to cough or to squeeze your pelvic muscles, as if you're trying to stop your urine stream or trying to stop passage of gas. If pelvic organ prolapse is suspected, you may be asked to repeat this test while sitting or standing. In these positions, the prolapse may become more pronounced.

To complete your internal examination, your uterus and ovaries may be examined for abnormal masses. This is generally done by inserting two gloved fingers into your vagina and pressing down on your abdomen with the other hand.

Digital rectal exam

Your provider inserts a gloved finger into your rectum to check for any masses or impacted stool, which may be contributing to urinary incontinence. A rectal exam can also help evaluate the strength of your pelvic floor muscles. To help determine muscle strength, your doctor may ask you to squeeze your anus around the examining finger, as if you're trying to avoid urinating or passing gas. Sometimes, a provider will also examine the tailbone (coccyx) during a digital rectal exam to check for pain or abnormal movement.

Male exam

In men, a physical exam may include examination of the penis, perineum, testicles, rectum and prostate gland.

Genital exam

Your penis and the area between your scrotum and anus (perineum) are examined. Chronic exposure to urine can cause skin problems on the foreskin, the head of the penis (glans penis) and the perineum. Sometimes this leads to swelling or enlargement of the penis. Each testicle also may be checked for indications of current or previous inflammation, which may be associated with urinary problems.

To test the nerves in your genital area, your provider may lightly stroke the perineal skin near your anus and watch or feel for an anal contraction. This reflex is sometimes called the anal wink. He or she may also lightly squeeze the glans penis and look for a similar anal contraction. This reflex is known as the bulbocavernosus reflex. If these reflexes aren't normal, it may mean that the nerves in your genital area are somehow contributing to your problem with urinary incontinence. These tests may feel a bit unusual, but they shouldn't be painful.

Digital rectal exam

For this exam, your provider inserts a gloved finger into your rectum to check the size, symmetry and texture of your prostate gland. If the gland is enlarged or infected, it may prevent your bladder from emptying completely, which may be causing your incontinence.

A digital rectal exam also provides an opportunity to check for any masses or impacted stool, which can contribute to urinary incontinence. The exam can also help demonstrate the strength of your pelvic floor muscles. To help determine the strength of these muscles, your doctor may ask you to squeeze your anus around the examining finger, as if you're trying to avoid urinating or passing gas. He or she may also examine the tailbone (coccyx) during a digital rectal exam to check for pain or abnormal movement.

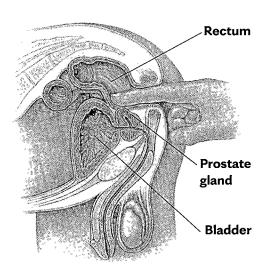

Rectum

Prostate gland

Bladder

During a male digital rectal examination, a doctor inserts a gloved, lubricated finger into the rectum and checks the size of the prostate gland. An enlarged gland may lead to incontinence.

SPECIFIC TESTS

Sometimes, the cause of urinary incontinence can be determined based solely on a physical examination. More often, though, additional information is needed to make a diagnosis. You may need to undergo one or more specialized tests. It's possible that you'll need just a few tests, such as a urinalysis and uroflowmetry. If they don't provide the expected results, additional testing may be necessary.

Urinalysis

Urinalysis is a routine test for urinary incontinence. A sample of your urine is sent to a laboratory, where it's checked for blood, glucose, bacteria or other abnormalities. For the sample to be collected, you're asked to urinate into a container.

Blood in your urine may indicate an irritation of your urinary tract, such as an infection, urinary stone or tumor. If you have blood in your urine, you may need to undergo another test to rule out the possibility of bladder cancer. This test, called urine cytology, specifically checks a urine sample for cancer cells.

If glucose is detected in your urine, you may have diabetes, which can increase your urine volume and make incontinence more likely. Additional testing can help confirm the diagnosis.

Bacteria in your urine can be a sign of a urinary tract infection. To get more information about the specific microbe causing the infection, your urine sample is sent to a laboratory to be cultured, called a urine culture test. If the culture is positive, you'll likely be prescribed a course of antibiotics.

Urodynamic testing

Urodynamic testing is any procedure that looks at how well the bladder, sphincters and urethra are storing and releasing urine. Most urodynamic tests focus on the bladder's ability to hold urine and empty itself steadily and completely. Urodynamic tests can also show whether the bladder is having involuntary contractions that cause urine leakage.

There are several different urodynamic tests that make up a urodynamic study. Your study may include one or more of the following tests:

Uroflowmetry

Uroflowmetry is a simple screening procedure that measures how fast your urine comes out — its speed and volume. The test is performed by having a person with a full bladder urinate into a special funnel that's connected to a measuring instrument. The measuring instrument calculates the amount of urine, rate of flow in seconds and length of time it takes to urinate.

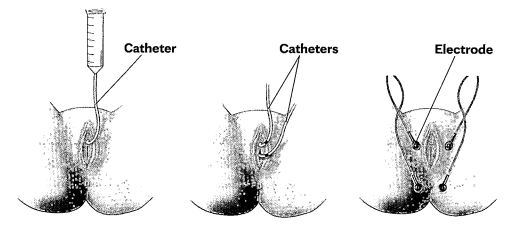

Catheter **Catheters** **Electrode**

Urodynamic tests monitor the urinary system in action. To determine how your bladder responds to pressure, it may be filled with water (left). For some of the tests, a catheter that senses changes in pressure is placed in the urethra and bladder while another pressure sensor is placed in the vagina or rectum (middle). In another test, small electrodes are placed on the skin near the urethra and rectum to record electrical activity of the pelvic floor muscles (right). This test can also be done on men.

The information is converted into a graph and interpreted by a doctor. It's used to help evaluate function of the lower urinary tract or help determine if there's an obstruction of normal urine outflow. If your peak or average flow rate is lower than normal, you may have an obstruction in your urethra or a weak bladder muscle.

Uroflowmetry measurements are noninvasive. They're generally performed in a doctor's office, and there's no anesthesia involved.

Postvoid residual test

Commonly referred to as the PVR test, this procedure helps determine whether you're having difficulty emptying your bladder. It measures the amount of urine left in your bladder in the five to 10 minutes after you urinate. A bladder that doesn't fully empty can lead to increased urinary frequency and can worsen stress incontinence.

For the test, you urinate into a specific container that measures your urine output. Your provider then checks the amount of remaining (residual) urine in your bladder in one of two ways.

One option is to insert a thin, soft tube (catheter) into your urethra and bladder to drain any remaining urine. This provides a clean sample for a urine culture and prepares you for additional tests, but the procedure is invasive and can be a bit uncomfortable. It also poses a small risk of urinary tract infection.

The other option for determining the amount of urine remaining in the bladder is to use ultrasound. For the test, a wandlike device (transducer) that sends out sound waves is placed over your abdomen and pelvic area. A computer transforms the sound waves into images of your bladder so that your doctor can see how full or empty it is. This option is quicker and less painful than catheterization. Plus, the ultrasound images can provide other important information about the overall condition and capacity of your bladder.

It's normal to have some urine remaining in your bladder. A normal PVR reading may be as high as 100 milliliters, or even higher among older adults. A reading over 250 milliliters or 25% of your total bladder capacity is generally considered abnormal. If your PVR reading is in this range after repeated tests, it may mean that you have an obstruction in your urinary tract or a problem with your bladder nerves or muscles.

Cystometry

A cystometry test measures the volume and pressure in your bladder — when it's at rest, as it fills with urine and as you urinate.

After your bladder is completely empty, a catheter is inserted into your urethra and bladder to measure the pressure. A small pressure monitor also may be inserted into the rectum or, in women, the vagina. A separate catheter is then used to fill your bladder with warm, sterile water. As your bladder fills, the pressure within your bladder is recorded. Normally, pressure increases by only very small amounts during filling. However, in some people with urinary incontinence, the bladder goes into spasms as it fills. This test also helps your doctor measure the strength of your bladder muscle.

During the test, you'll be asked when you first feel the urge to urinate and when that urge becomes strong. You'll also be asked at several points to cough or bear down. The bladder pressure at which you leak urine when you cough or strain is called the abdominal leak point pressure. At the end of the test, you urinate into a special device, with the pressure sensors still in place. This is known as a voiding pressure test. Last, the pressure-sensing catheter will be slowly drawn through your urethra to measure the urethra's ability to close. This part of the test is called the urethral pressure profile.

After the test, you may need to go to the bathroom often and the need may be urgent. Your urine may be slightly pink for about a day. If these problems persist or you develop signs of infection, call your provider.

Leak point pressure measurement

This test, generally combined with a cystometry test, measures the pressure in your bladder at the point of leakage. While the bladder is being filled for the cystometry test, it may suddenly contract and squeeze some water out without warning. A special device (manometer)

measures the pressure inside the bladder when this leakage occurs.

This reading may provide information about the kind of bladder problem that exists. You may be asked to apply pressure to your bladder by coughing, shifting position, or exhaling while holding your nose and mouth. These actions help determine if the sphincter muscles are functioning normally.

Pressure flow study

This study measures the amount of bladder pressure needed for you to urinate and the rate of urine flow that a specific pressure generates. You empty your bladder, during which time a manometer measures your bladder pressure and flow rate. A pressure flow study helps identify bladder outlet blockage, a condition that men can experience with prostate enlargement.

Bladder outlet blockage is less common in women but can occur in certain conditions, such as when the bladder bulges into the vagina, called a prolapsed bladder (cystocele).

Electromyography

Electromyography (EMG) uses special sensors to measure the electrical activity of the muscles and nerves in and around the bladder and sphincters. This test may be done if nerve or muscle damage may be causing your incontinence and your doctor wants to know if the bladder and urethra are working in a coordinated fashion.

Small adhesive electrode patches are placed on the skin near your urethra and rectum. A machine then records the electrical current created when your pelvic floor muscles contract.

Video urodynamic tests

Video urodynamic tests take pictures and videos of the bladder while it's filling and emptying. Some other names for these tests include cystogram or voiding cystourethrogram.

Video urodynamic tests may use X-rays or ultrasound. If X-ray equipment is used, the bladder will be filled with a special fluid, called a contrast medium, that shows up on X-rays. As the fluid moves through your urinary tract and out of your body when you urinate, a series of X-ray images is taken. If ultrasound equipment is used, the bladder is filled with warm water and sound waves create pictures of the bladder.

The pictures and videos obtained during urodynamic testing show the size and shape of the bladder, and they outline the urinary tract, indicating abnormalities or obstructions. Video urodynamic tests may be done in conjunction with uroflowmetry, cystometry or both.

There can be some discomfort when the catheter is inserted into the bladder to fill it with a contrast medium or warm water. Therefore, a local anesthesia may be administered beforehand. After the test, you may have some pain while urinating and your urine might be slightly pink. If these problems persist or you develop signs of infection, call your provider.

Cystoscopy

Cystoscopy allows a doctor to see the inside of your urethra and bladder (see page 52). A thin tube with a tiny lens (cystoscope) is inserted into your urethra and bladder, and your bladder is filled with sterile fluid to stretch the bladder. This offers a better view of your bladder wall.

During a cystoscopy exam, your doctor checks the bladder and urethra for potential causes of urinary incontinence. Bladder infections, tumors, abscesses, stones and other abnormalities can cause urinary incontinence. Other contributing factors can include problems with the urethra, such as pouches or sac openings (urethral diverticula) or urethral narrowing caused by scar tissue or an obstructing prostate gland (urethral stricture).

During the procedure, your doctor may remove a sample of bladder tissue for lab analysis or even remove a small stone.

Cystoscopy typically takes about 15 to 20 minutes from start to finish. You're usually given a local anesthetic and you remain awake during the procedure. You may feel some discomfort and the need to urinate as your bladder fills.

After the test, your urethra may be sore and you may feel a mild burning when you urinate. You may also see small amounts of blood in your urine. These problems usually go away within a few days. If the problems persist or you develop signs or symptoms of infection, including cloudy urine, fever or chills, contact your medical provider.

CT urogram

A computerized tomography (CT) urogram is an imaging exam to evaluate your urinary tract, including your kidneys, bladder and the tubes (ureters) that carry urine from your kidneys to your bladder.

CT urography uses X-rays to generate multiple images of a slice of the area in your body being studied, including bones, soft tissues and blood vessels. These images are then sent to a computer and quickly reconstructed into very detailed 2D images.

For this test, you usually lie on your back on an exam table, though you may be asked to lie on your side or your stomach. Straps and pillows may be used to help you maintain the correct position and help keep you still. During the procedure you may be asked to change positions.

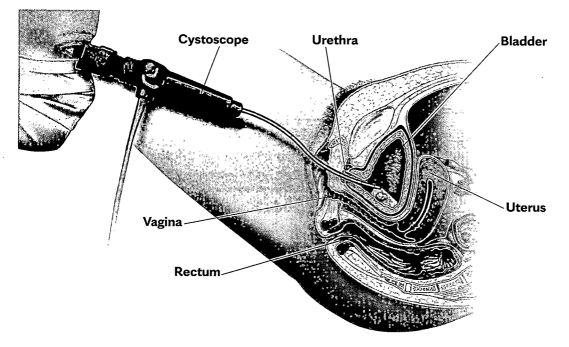

Cystoscopic examination allows your doctor to see inside your urethra and bladder. It can help in diagnosing urethral and bladder problems that cause urinary incontinence.

An intravenous (IV) line will be placed into a vein in your hand or arm through which the X-ray dye will be injected. The dye flows into your kidneys, ureters and bladder, outlining each of these structures. X-ray pictures are taken at specific times during the exam so your doctor can clearly see your urinary tract and assess how well it's working or look for any abnormalities. You may feel a warm, flushed sensation when the dye is injected and sense a metallic taste in your mouth for a minute or two.

Once you're ready, the exam table will move quickly through the scanner to determine the correct starting position. For the actual scans, the table will move slowly through the machine while the images are taken. If needed, the machine may make several passes.

Other tests

Additional tests sometimes performed to help make a diagnosis include an ultrasound examination, a CT scan and magnetic resonance imaging (MRI) of the pelvic area. These tests look at other parts of your urinary tract or genitals and check for possible abnormalities that may be contributing to your bladder problems.

DETERMINING YOUR TREATMENT

After your diagnostic tests are complete, your provider will review the information he or she has collected from the tests, as well as from your medical history and physical examination. From this informa-

tion, your doctor diagnoses the type of incontinence you have and how best to treat it. The course of treatment recommended will depend on a number of factors. In addition to the type of incontinence you have, the severity of your symptoms and your age, overall physical health and lifestyle are other factors taken into consideration.

If your provider thinks conservative therapies may be effective, he or she may recommend that you start them. Conservative therapies don't involve surgery. They include behavioral techniques such as bladder training, scheduled toilet trips, pelvic floor muscle (Kegel) exercises, and managing the amount of fluids you drink and when you drink them.

Medications are another form of conservative therapy. For some forms of incontinence, medications can be helpful. They work in several ways, including helping to calm overactive muscles and nerves, relax the bladder muscle, improve urinary flow or decrease urine production. Conservative therapies also include medical devices that may help prevent leakage or support the bladder.

It's possible that your provider may recommend a combination of therapies, which are discussed in detail in upcoming chapters. If conservative therapies aren't effective or aren't an option, surgery may be considered.

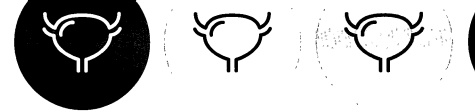
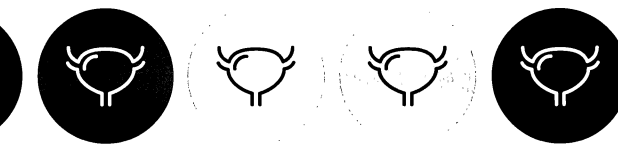
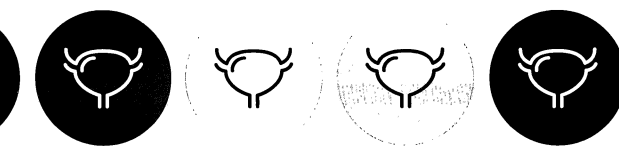
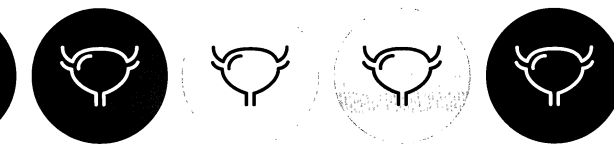
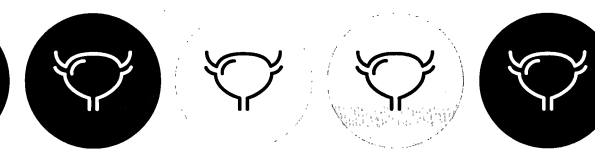
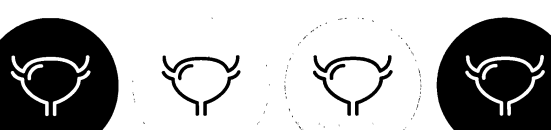

4

Conservative treatments

There are a variety of treatments for urinary incontinence. The one that's best for you depends on the type of incontinence you have, your sex, and how much incontinence affects your daily life.

Most doctors and other medical providers begin with conservative treatments that are noninvasive or minimally invasive and have proven benefits, little risk and few side effects. If this approach doesn't work, you and your provider may consider additional care, including medication or more-invasive procedures, such as surgery.

This chapter covers noninvasive and minimally invasive treatments that can improve urinary incontinence. The therapies are generally safe, easy and relatively inexpensive. Your medical provider may suggest trying one or more of these approaches as a first line of treatment.

LIFESTYLE CHANGES

It's possible that changes in your daily routine may be the only treatment required to manage your incontinence. Your provider may suggest that you experiment with lifestyle changes before trying other types of treatment to see if some fairly easy modifications can reduce your symptoms.

Fluid and diet management

How much and what types of fluid you drink each day, as well as the types of food

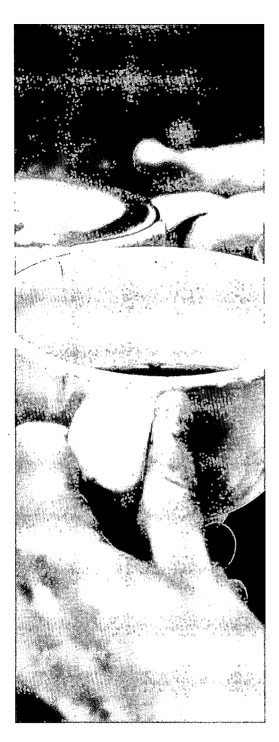

you eat, may have an influence on your bladder habits. Too much or too little fluid can trigger an overactive bladder, in which your bladder spasms and sends messages to your brain that it's full even when it's not. This can give you a strong urge to urinate or make you want to urinate more often, sometimes causing leakage.

Occasionally, certain foods can irritate the bladder and increase urinary frequency, urgency and leakage.

Too much fluid

It's true that drinking too much fluid can make you urinate more often. If you drink a lot of fluid at a given time, the excess fluid can overwhelm your bladder and create a strong sense of urgency. If you exercise a lot or work outdoors on a regular basis, you may need to take in additional fluids. But rather than drink a large amount at once, try to spread your fluid consumption throughout the day.

If you get up several times a night to urinate, try to drink most of your fluids in the morning and afternoon and eliminate alcohol and caffeinated beverages. The recommended fluid intake is approximately 60 ounces daily. Another way to think of it is drinking eight 8-ounce glasses — the 8x8 rule. But not everyone needs this much fluid. Some people can get by with less. If you exercise or work outdoors on a regular basis, you may need additional fluids.

Remember that your fluids can come from any beverage you drink, not just water, and also from foods, such as soup or fruit. If you need to go to the bathroom often and also experience urgent needs to go, aim for at least half of the fluids you consume to be plain water to reduce irritation to the lining of the bladder.

Too little fluid

Surprisingly, drinking too little fluid also can cause problems. Too little fluid can cause your urine to become overly concentrated with your body's waste products.

Highly concentrated urine is dark yellow in color and has a strong smell. Concentrated urine can irritate your bladder, increasing the urge and frequency with which you need to go. It may also put you at risk of a urinary tract infection, which can in itself cause symptoms of urge incontinence.

Bladder irritants

Certain foods and beverages can irritate your bladder as well. Caffeine and alcohol both act as diuretics, which means that they increase urine production. This can lead to increased frequency and urgency.

Consuming too many acidic fruits and fruit juices (orange, grapefruit, lemon, lime), spicy foods, tomato-based products, carbonated drinks, and foods that contain artificial sweeteners also may irritate your bladder. Why these foods sometimes cause irritation isn't exactly understood.

If caffeine or alcohol or one of these other foods is a regular part of your diet, you might try eliminating it for about a week to see if your symptoms improve. Cut out only one food or beverage at a time so that you can tell which one might be causing the problem. You may not have to eliminate your favorite foods entirely. Simply cut down on the amount you consume and see if that helps. See page 176 for a more complete list of foods and beverages that can cause bladder irritation.

Other lifestyle changes

Other changes in your daily habits may also improve symptoms of incontinence. These include changing or reducing problem medications, managing your weight, getting more physical activity, stopping smoking if you smoke, and treating constipation.

Changing your medications

Medications that you're taking for another medical condition may be causing or contributing to your incontinence. Talk to your doctor about your medications. If your doctor thinks that a drug you're taking may be contributing to your problems, he or she may suggest an alternative dosage or another drug that may not cause these kinds of side effects.

Examples of medications that may contribute to incontinence include high blood pressure drugs, heart medications, diuretics, muscle relaxants, sedatives and antidepressants. Common effects of these medications include:

- Relaxation of the urethral muscle, which can lead to leakage
- Relaxation of the bladder muscle, which can lead to urinary retention and overflow incontinence
- Diminished awareness of the need to urinate
- Overproduction of urine, which can overwhelm an already stressed bladder
- Constipation, which can obstruct urine flow and aggravate an overactive bladder
- Chronic coughing, which can worsen stress incontinence

See page 178 for a list of medications that can contribute to urinary problems.

Managing your weight

Being overweight can contribute to urinary incontinence, particularly stress and mixed incontinence. This may be because excessive body weight increases pressure on your abdomen during physical activity, which, in turn, may increase pressure on your bladder and affect the ability of your urethra to shift position during activity. The result is urine leakage.

In studies of overweight adults, results indicate that individuals who are obese have a higher risk of incontinence than do individuals at a normal weight. Studies have also found that weight loss can improve symptoms. If you're overweight and you're experiencing urinary inconti-

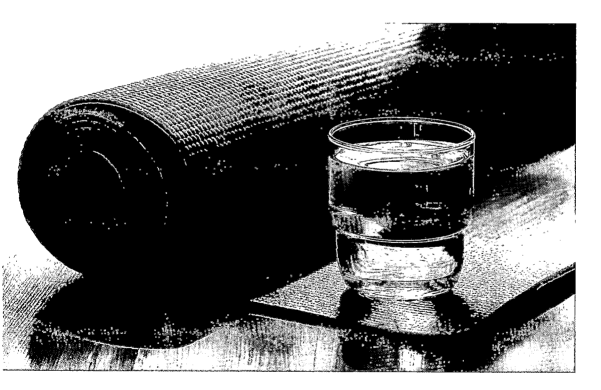

nence, taking steps to lose weight may be one way to help treat your incontinence.

Getting more physical activity

Physical activity is an important aspect of a healthy lifestyle. In general, all adults should get at least 150 minutes of moderate physical activity each week. Studies show that more physical activity is also associated with reduced urinary incontinence.

Stopping smoking

Tobacco use is another lifestyle factor that may have an impact on urinary incontinence. Heavy smokers in particular often develop a severe chronic cough, which can place added pressure on the bladder and aggravate urinary incontinence.

Stopping smoking allows your lungs to regain some normalcy, thereby reducing or even eliminating your coughing and its effects on your bladder. Quitting smoking also provides numerous other health benefits.

BEHAVIOR AND PHYSICAL THERAPIES

The following therapies can be helpful for individuals experiencing mild to moderate symptoms in which lifestyle changes alone aren't enough. The practices may also be used in combination with medications or minimally invasive procedures.

Bladder training

With an overactive bladder, you may become accustomed to urinating frequently or going at the slightest urge. Sometimes, you may go to the bathroom even if you don't have the urge to urinate because you want to avoid a possible accident. In time, your bladder begins sending "full" messages to your brain even when it's not full, and you feel compelled to go.

Typically, a person urinates five to six times a day, with the bladder holding as much as 2 cups of urine. In the case of an overactive bladder, you may go to the bathroom more than eight to 10 times daily — and more than twice a night — each time urinating only a small amount.

Bladder training involves teaching your bladder new habits by urinating on a set schedule. This makes it possible for you to gain control over frequent urges and allows your bladder enough time to fill up properly.

Bladder training can be helpful for men and women who have urge and other types of incontinence. It may also involve double voiding — urinating, then waiting a few minutes and trying again. This exercise can help you empty your bladder more completely to avoid overflow incontinence.

A bladder training program may be used alone or in combination with other therapies. It usually involves the following basic steps.

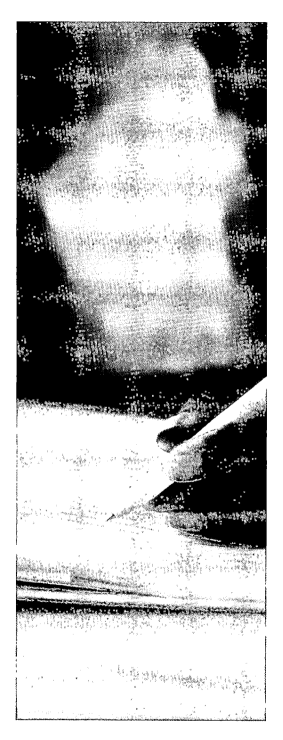

Identify your pattern

For a few days, record in a bladder diary (see page 174) every time you urinate. For example, you may find that you tend to urinate every hour on the hour. Your doctor can use the information in your diary to help you establish a schedule for your bladder training.

Set your bathroom intervals

After you've discovered how much time typically passes between bathroom breaks, your doctor may suggest that you extend that interval by 15 minutes. So, if you determine that your usual interval is one hour, you work to extend that interval to an hour and 15 minutes.

Stick to your schedule

Once you've established a daytime schedule — you probably won't need to follow a schedule at night — do your best to stick to it. Begin your schedule by urinating immediately after you wake up in the morning. After that, if an urge arises but it's not time for you to go, try as hard as you can to wait it out. If you feel that you're going to have an accident, go to the bathroom but then return to your preset schedule.

Urges typically build to a peak and then gradually diminish. Responding immediately to an urge by rushing to the bathroom only serves to increase your sense of urgency, and it may invite an accident. Instead, stop and take a deep breath.

When you have an urge, relax and try to think of something other than going to the bathroom. Play a mind game such as recalling the last three books you've read or the movies you've been meaning to watch. It may help to do five to 10 quick, strong pelvic floor muscle contractions (described on page 179) to help alleviate the urge and maintain control. If you feel an urge to go at your scheduled time, stop and wait until the urge recedes, then proceed to the bathroom.

Increase your intervals

Your goal is to gradually lengthen the time between trips to the bathroom until you reach intervals of two to four hours.

You might do this by extending the time between bathroom trips by an additional 15 minutes each week until you reach your desired goal.

Don't be discouraged if you don't succeed the first few times. Keep practicing, and your ability to maintain control is likely to improve. See page 181 for instructions on performing timed voiding drills.

Pelvic floor muscle training

This form of treatment involves doing exercises commonly referred to as Kegels to strengthen weak urethral sphincter and pelvic floor muscles — the muscles that help control urination and defecation.

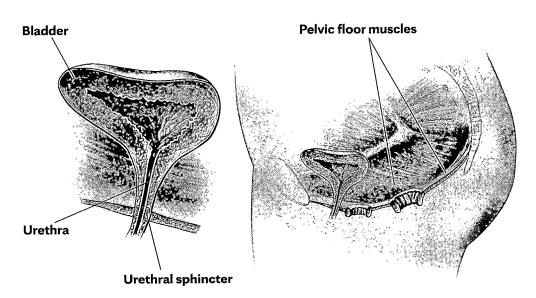

Bladder

Urethra

Urethral sphincter

Pelvic floor muscles

Pelvic floor muscle exercises involve squeezing and relaxing the muscles in the pelvic and genital area. Strengthening these muscles can help improve bladder control.

The pelvic floor muscles serve dual roles. One is to open and close the urethra and anus. The other is to support the bladder and rectum as you exert yourself while doing such things as walking, lifting and sneezing. The pelvic floor muscles lie at the bottom of your pelvis and attach to the front, back and sides of your pelvic bone.

For women, the correct way to perform pelvic floor muscle exercises involves a combination of two things — a squeeze around the urethra, vagina and anus, and a lift of the muscles inward and up toward your head. For men, activating the muscles as if retracting the penis is an effective way to do these exercises.

Some women use vaginal cones to assist with pelvic floor muscle training. These cones are small weights that are inserted into the vagina. You hold the weights in place using your pelvic floor muscles. As you're ready, you progress to the next vaginal cone with a higher weight.

Your doctor may recommend that you perform pelvic floor muscle exercises three or four times a day to help treat your incontinence. The exercises are especially effective for women with stress incontinence, but they can also reduce or eliminate urge incontinence. See page 179 for information about how to perform pelvic floor exercises.

PRODUCTS AND DEVICES

A number of products and devices can help reduce the frequency, severity or potential embarrassment of urinary incontinence. These items may be used to help manage your condition or to keep you dry while waiting for other treatments to take effect. Some of these devices are just for women, some just for men, and some can be used by both.

Absorption products

As their name suggests, absorption products are designed to absorb urine that leaks from your bladder, keeping your skin and clothing dry.

Absorbent pads

Various absorbent pads help manage urine loss. Most absorbent products are no more bulky than normal underwear, and you can wear them easily under everyday clothing. Men who have problems with dribbles of urine can use a drip collector — a small pocket of absorbent padding that's worn over the penis and held in place by close-fitting underwear.

Other types of absorbent products include adult diapers, pads or panty liners. These items can be purchased at drugstores, supermarkets and medical supply stores.

Absorption collection system

This is a relatively new noninvasive device for women. It includes a small external catheter that's positioned between the labia and buttocks. The catheter contains soft material and a low-pressure vacuum that gently draws urine away from the body, keeping your skin dry. The device can be used when lying down or seated, including at night while sleeping.

Thin, flexible tubing connects the catheter to a small storage container. Urine absorbed by the catheter is gathered in the container, which you empty after each use. For women who leak considerable urine at night, the collection system may be an alternative to having to make multiple adult diaper changes, causing disrupted sleep.

Female inserts

Inserts are intended just for women. The benefit of inserts is that you control their use — you might wear an insert all of the time or just during certain activities. Although they don't cure incontinence, they can help you manage it. The downside is that, for some women, an insert can be uncomfortable and may even be painful. Your doctor can help you decide if an insert would be helpful for you.

Urethral inserts

Urethral inserts are small, tampon-like disposable devices (plugs) that you insert into your urethra to prevent urine from leaking out. Urethral inserts aren't for everyday use because they can cause irritation. They generally work best for women who have predictable leakage during certain activities, such as while jogging or playing tennis. You insert the device before an activity. When the activity is complete or you need to urinate, you simply remove the plug.

Urethral inserts are available by prescription. They're generally made of soft silicone and have a tube shape with a balloon-like tip at one end and a flange at the other.

The device is inserted into the urethra with an applicator. Because the balloon tip is soft and filled with fluid, it conforms to the shape of your urethra and bladder and creates a seal around your bladder neck, preventing urine from leaking out. To remove a urethral insert, you grasp the flange, which remains on the outside of your urethra, and pull the device out.

Vaginal inserts

Vaginal inserts — also known as urethral support inserts — are similar to urethral inserts, but the devices are inserted into the vagina instead of the urethra. When placed in the vagina, the device lifts and supports the urethra.

There are a couple of different types — an absorbent, disposable insert that's available without a prescription and a nondisposable insert that requires a prescription. You insert the disposable product into your vagina with an applicator, similar to a tampon, and remove and dispose of it when it needs to be changed.

The nondisposable type comes in various sizes and is made of silicone and shaped

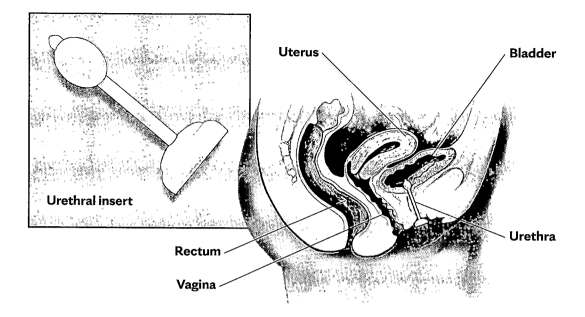

Urethral insert

Uterus

Bladder

Rectum

Vagina

Urethra

A urethral insert is placed in the female urethra where it forms a barrier between the bladder and the outside, preventing leakage of urine during activities that might cause incontinence.

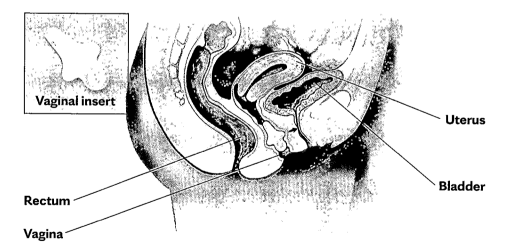

Vaginal insert

Uterus

Bladder

Rectum

Vagina

A vaginal insert is placed in the female vagina, where it provides support to the bladder neck and urethra, helping to prevent urine leakage.

like a bell or small plug. You gently insert the device into your vagina, and after each use you clean it with soap and warm water. You can use the same insert for up to a year.

Some women use vaginal inserts only during activities that require increased support, such as during exercise and when traveling. Others use them the entire day.

Because urethral support inserts are placed in the vagina instead of the urethra, women generally find them more comfortable. However, there's greater chance of experiencing some leakage when using a vaginal insert than when using a urethral insert.

Pessaries

On occasion a doctor may recommend a pessary. This is a silicone or latex device, usually shaped like a ring or a dish, that's inserted into your vagina and that you can wear all day. You may benefit from a pessary if you have incontinence due to a dropped (prolapsed) bladder or uterus.

A pessary requires a prescription, and it's usually fitted and put in place by a doctor. If you have an infection in your pelvic area, it must be treated before you're fitted with the device, to avoid complications. You should be able to urinate with a pessary in place if it's fitted correctly. You do need to remove it regularly to clean it.

Side effects can include an allergic reaction to the latex or silicone, infection,

irritation, and pressure sores. Pressure sores are more common if you're post-menopausal, most likely because vaginal tissue is typically more sensitive and less elastic after menopause. Vaginal estrogen cream may be used to help avoid this.

Male compression products

The idea behind these products is to prevent or reduce urine leakage by providing compression to the penis. Several different types of cuffs or clamps are available that fit over the end of the penis. You adjust the tightness to stop the flow of urine. These devices come in different sizes for improved fit.

Talk to your doctor about how to best use compression products. Some devices shouldn't be worn for more than two to three hours at a time. If left on for too long, they can cause tissue damage, swelling and pain. Newer products may be worn for longer periods.

Biofeedback

Biofeedback can help with pelvic floor muscle exercises, particularly if you're having trouble feeling or sensing these muscles. Biofeedback is a system that uses a variety of monitoring procedures and equipment to provide you with feedback on bodily responses, such as your muscle activity, heart rate, skin temperature and brain activity. Using this information, you can learn to control some of these bodily responses to improve your health.

In the case of urinary incontinence, biofeedback may be used to monitor the electrical activity of your pelvic floor muscles. This is done to make sure that you're using the right muscles when doing the exercises. Many trained specialists conduct biofeedback sessions. These specialists include occupational therapists, physical therapists, nurses and psychologists. In addition, there are biofeedback devices you can use at home.

During a biofeedback session, a therapist applies electrode sensors to the skin area near the anus and vagina in females. Sometimes, the therapist inserts a small sensor into the female vagina or the male rectum. Sensors may be placed in both the vagina and rectum in women. If a sensor can't be placed internally, small electrodes are used instead and placed on the skin adjacent to the pelvic floor muscles. Electrodes may also be placed on your abdomen, thighs or buttocks to see if you're unintentionally using these muscles during a pelvic floor muscle contraction.

You're then asked to contract your pelvic floor muscles several times as the sensors register the strength and control of your contractions. By watching the readout and comparing your response with the ideal response, you can modify your contractions so that you're doing the exercises properly.

Devices you use at home to measure the strength of your pelvic floor muscle contractions can be purchased at drugstores, medical supply stores and online. Not all of them require a prescription.

Some of the devices also include an app that provides real-time visual feedback so that you can see if you're exercising correctly. If you're interested in using biofeedback at home, talk to your doctor or a therapist and ask if such a device might be appropriate for you.

Electrical stimulation

Weak electrical current is sometimes used to treat the muscles and nerves that play a role in urinary storage and voiding. The current is applied through electrodes that are placed either near the muscles or directly into the nerves.

Pelvic floor muscle stimulation

If your pelvic floor muscles are weak or you need help performing pelvic floor muscle exercises, your doctor or therapist might suggest electrical pelvic stimulation. With electrical stimulation, electrodes may be placed on the skin near the anus. Or a probe with electrodes, similar to the one used during biofeedback, may be inserted into the rectum or vagina to gently stimulate and strengthen your pelvic floor muscles.

The electrical stimulation causes your pelvic floor muscles to contract without effort on your part (passive contractions). Electrical stimulation can also be used with strengthening exercises.

This technique can be effective for stress and urge incontinence in both men and women, but multiple treatments may be necessary to achieve maximum benefit. However, each treatment often brings improvement. Electrical stimulation may be done in your doctor's or therapist's office, or you can do it at home with a portable battery-operated device.

Among women, another way to receive electrical stimulation is by wearing a garment, similar to bicycle shorts, that contains electrodes in the fabric. The garment is worn about 30 minutes a day, and some women notice a decrease in bladder leakage in two to three months.

Tibial nerve stimulation

Inspired by acupuncture, this method of electrical stimulation is used specifically to treat urge incontinence. Rather than stimulating the pelvic muscles, it stimulates the tibial nerve located in your lower leg. The tibial nerve is connected to the sacral nerve group, which plays a direct role in regulating bladder contractions. Stimulation of the tibial nerve can help moderate imbalanced nerve messages an overactive bladder sends to the brain, reducing bladder contractions and symptoms of urgency and frequency.

Tibial nerve stimulation may be done in your doctor's office. During the procedure, a thin needle is inserted just above your anklebone. Low-frequency electrical stimulation is passed through the needle to your tibial nerve for approximately 30 minutes.

The procedure is painless, but you might notice your toes spread out or your big toe curl. You may also feel a sensation spread through the sole of your foot. The stimulation is applied once a week for about three months and then as needed thereafter, depending on your response to the therapy.

Preliminary clinical trials indicate the therapy may substantially improve signs and symptoms of incontinence, particularly frequency and urgency. More studies are needed to examine the therapy's long-term effects. Tibial nerve stimulation may provide an alternative for people who would rather not have surgery and in which other conservative therapies haven't been successful.

Sacral nerve stimulation

Direct stimulation of the sacral nerve, which branches off your lower spinal cord, is another option for treating an overactive bladder. This therapy requires a surgical procedure and is discussed in Chapter 6.

Catheters

If other therapies fail or are unacceptable, or if you need help while waiting for treatment such as surgery, your doctor may recommend use of a catheter. A catheter is a thin tube that's inserted in the urethra. It allows urine to drain from the bladder. Side effects of catheter use can include urinary tract infections and skin irritation. Proper sterilization techniques can help prevent these problems from occurring.

Catheter types and techniques include:

- *Intermittent self-catheterization.* A medical provider teaches you how to drain your bladder using self-catheterization. The process involves inserting a thin, flexible tube through your urethra and into your bladder, allowing urine to drain out. You also are provided information on how many times a day to perform self-catheterization. Self-catheterization can be useful for individuals who cannot completely empty their bladders or need to irrigate their bladders.

- *Indwelling catheter.* Also called a Foley catheter, this type of catheter remains in place continuously. The end of the catheter has a balloon that's inflated with sterile water after the end is inserted inside the bladder. The inflated balloon prevents the catheter from slipping out. Urinary tract infections are more likely to occur with long-term use of an indwelling catheter than with intermittent self-catheterization.

- *Condom catheter.* This is a special condom that fits over the male penis and is attached to a tube that collects

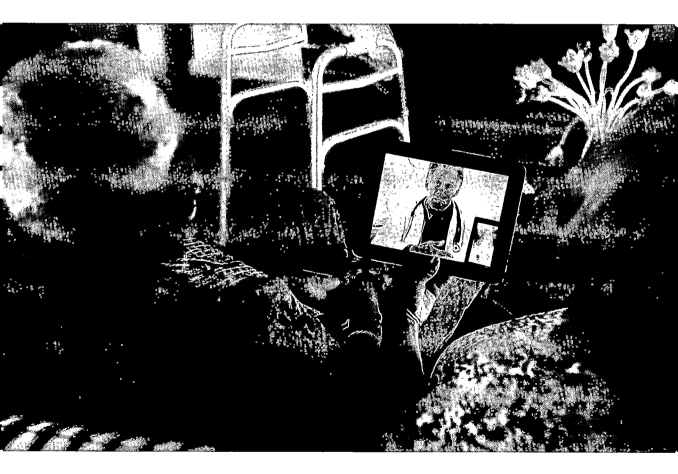

urine. Condom catheters come in disposable and reusable forms. An advantage of the condom catheter is that it doesn't require an internal catheter to be placed in your urethra. As a result, urinary tract infections are less common, although skin irritation may occur due to friction between the catheter and your penis. Condom catheters are only for short-term use because of the risk of side effects.

YOUR ROLE

The behavior changes, procedures and devices discussed in this chapter can be very effective in treating urinary incontinence, and many provide substantial benefits with minimal side effects. Doctors and other medical professionals can help you in many ways — by teaching you how to use the different therapies and providing you with feedback — but you play a vital role in your treatment.

Once you begin a bladder training program, for example, or learn how to do pelvic floor muscle exercises, your job is to actively carry out your prescribed treatment. Many people perform pelvic floor muscle exercises incorrectly. Therefore, you might benefit from seeing a physical or occupational therapist who can teach you the correct performance of the pelvic floor muscle contraction and relaxation for pelvic floor muscle training.

Keep in mind that behavior therapies such as bladder training and pelvic floor muscle exercises take some time and practice before you begin to see results.

But persistence pays off. If you stick with the program, you'll more than likely begin to see an improvement in your symptoms.

If one type of therapy doesn't work, talk with your provider about other options. Just because one treatment may not work, doesn't mean that others won't be effective. Often, a combination of treatments works best.

Finally, try to surround yourself with a positive network of family and friends. Although incontinence may be an embarrassing topic to discuss at first, you might be surprised at how common it really is. You may also discover how understanding others can be once they learn the implications of the condition and the benefits of its treatment, both for you and for them.

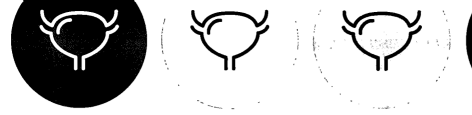
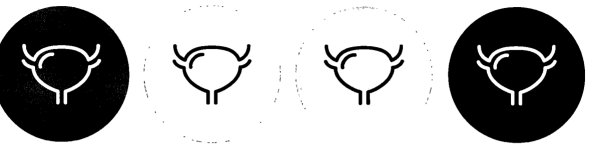
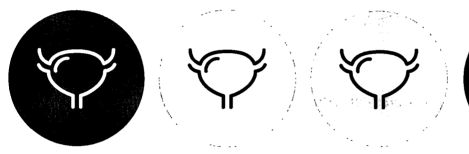
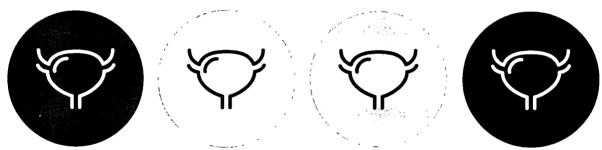
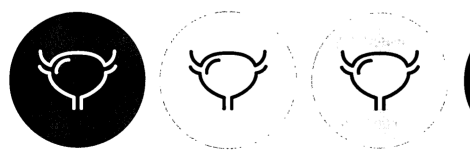
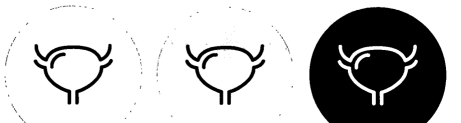

5

Medications and injections

In some cases, medications may improve symptoms of urinary incontinence. Medications are most effective for urge and mixed incontinence, and they may be prescribed in conjunction with conservative therapies, such as bladder training. Medications aren't used to treat stress incontinence.

Injections of substances into specific tissues or muscles are another option for some individuals. Botulinum toxin type A (Botox) blocks the actions of an overactive bladder muscle. Bulking agents add bulk to tissues surrounding the urethra, helping to prevent urine leakage.

Whether you're a candidate for a medication or an injection and the type you receive will depend on the type of incontinence you have and your symptoms.

MEDICATIONS

As mentioned in the previous chapter, the first step in treating stress or urge incontinence is with lifestyle changes and behavior therapy, which may include pelvic floor muscle training and timed voiding. Medications, when used in combination with other treatments, may help improve symptoms and reduce or eliminate leakage.

Medications are generally most helpful for people with urge incontinence from an overactive bladder. There are currently no medications to treat stress incontinence. This is partly because behavior therapy often produces satisfactory results and because few medications have shown promise in treating stress incontinence. However, newer medications are being studied and may become available in the future.

If your doctor is considering medication to treat your incontinence, it's important that he or she knows about all of the drugs you currently take. Medications taken for other illnesses, including over-the-counter drugs or herbal remedies, can interact with incontinence medications, possibly worsening your symptoms. To avoid such an interaction, your doctor needs to be aware of all of your medications.

Anticholinergics

If you could closely examine the cells in your body, you would see tiny receptors on the outside surface of each cell. These receptors act as gateways for various chemical messengers (neurotransmitters) from the brain that tell your cells how to act. Each neurotransmitter fits a matching receptor, like a key in a lock.

Acetylcholine is a neurotransmitter that acts on bladder muscle cells causing the bladder to contract. An overactive bladder is characterized by abnormal contractions, which make you want to urinate even when your bladder isn't full. Anticholinergic drugs help calm an overactive bladder by blocking the receptors to which acetylcholine normally binds. This action decreases involuntary bladder muscle contractions, reduces the strength of the involuntary contractions and increases the storage capacity of your bladder. As a result, your urgency, frequency and incontinence episodes are diminished.

Several drugs fall under this category. They include the medications oxybutynin (Ditropan XL), tolterodine (Detrol, Detrol LA), darifenacin (Enablex), fesoterodine (Toviaz), solifenacin (Vesicare, Vesicare LS) and trospium.

Two of the most commonly prescribed anticholinergics are oxybutynin and tolterodine. Both are available in an extended-release form, which has two advantages over the immediate-release forms. You only need to take them once a day instead of several times a day, and they have fewer side effects.

Extended-release forms of oxybutynin and tolterodine are thought to be similarly effective. The immediate-release form of the drug may still be helpful if you experience incontinence only at certain times, such as at night.

Oxybutynin is also available as a skin patch (Gelnique, Oxytrol) that delivers a continuous amount of medication to your body for at least three days. Studies have found the skin patch to be as effective as the immediate-release oxybutynin in pill form, but with fewer side effects.

Anticholinergics are often the drugs of choice for women with urge incontinence from an overactive bladder. They're also used in men with an overactive bladder. In men, sometimes symptoms of urge incontinence are the result of an enlarged prostate gland (benign prostatic hyperplasia, or BPH), but many times they're not. Your doctor will help determine the cause and which treatment option is best for you.

Regular use of anticholinergic medications could lead to dementia. That's the takeaway message from a recent long-term study published in the *Journal of the American Medical Association*. Researchers studying approximately 3,500 individuals age 65 and older found that those who took anticholinergic medications for more than three years were at greater risk of dementia.

Anticholinergic medications block the action of acetylcholine, a substance that transmits messages in your nervous system. In the brain, acetylcholine is involved in learning and memory. In the rest of the body, it stimulates muscle contractions. In addition to medications to control an overactive bladder, anticholinergic medications include tricyclic antidepressants, antipsychotic medications, drugs that relieve the symptoms of Parkinson's disease and drugs taken to control epileptic seizures.

When the researchers studied anticholinergic medications and their uses, they found that people who used these medications were more likely to have developed dementia than those who didn't use them. And they found that dementia risk increased along with the cumulative dose. Individuals taking anticholinergic medications for an equivalent of three years or more had a 54% higher risk of dementia than people who took the same dose for three months or less.

Results of the study suggest that doctors should exercise caution when prescribing these medications to middle-aged and older adults, especially if better alternatives exist.

When urge incontinence is associated with an enlarged prostate gland, sometimes the first step is to treat the prostate enlargement. Other times, a doctor may recommend treating the incontinence first.

Side effects and cautions

The most common side effect of anticholinergics is dry mouth. To counteract this effect, you might suck on a piece of candy or chew gum to produce more saliva. Other less common side effects include constipation, heartburn, blurry vision, urinary retention, and cognitive side effects such as dizziness and confusion.

The most common side effect of the oxybutynin skin patch is skin irritation. Your doctor may recommend rotating the location of the patch to reduce irritation.

You shouldn't take an anticholinergic medication if you have problems with urinary retention — you have trouble starting your urine flow or emptying your bladder. This type of medication also isn't recommended if you have uncontrolled narrow-angle glaucoma or a gastrointestinal obstruction. Anticholinergics should be used with caution if you have liver or kidney problems.

Beta-3 adrenergic agonists

Mirabegron (Myrbetriq) belongs to a class of medications known as beta-3 adrenergic agonists. This extended-release tablet taken once daily improves the storage capacity of the bladder by relaxing the bladder muscle during filling. It's thought to be as effective as other medications for treating urge incontinence.

Side effects and cautions

Side effects include irritation of the nose and pharynx, constipation, and hypertension. The drug isn't recommended if you have moderate to severe kidney or liver disease or uncontrolled high blood pressure.

Alpha-adrenergic blockers

These drugs were originally developed to treat high blood pressure and are also used to treat prostate enlargement in men. They may be an option for men with symptoms of urge and overflow incontinence that's associated with BPH.

Alpha-adrenergic blockers, also known as alpha blockers, promote the relaxation of smooth muscle found in the bladder neck and urethra. They do this by blocking the neurotransmitter norepinephrine from binding with alpha-adrenergic receptors in these areas. The result is increased urine flow and possibly a decrease in the number of times you need to urinate.

Your doctor may recommend one of these drugs if you're having symptoms of overactive bladder associated with an enlarged prostate gland. Examples of alpha-adrenergic blockers include tamsulosin (Flomax), alfuzosin (Uroxatral), doxazosin (Cardura, Cardura XL), silodosin (Rapaflo) and terazosin.

Side effects and cautions

Alpha-adrenergic blockers can cause a sudden drop in blood pressure when you change from one position to another, such as getting up from bed or standing up from a chair (postural hypotension). This tends to be particularly true if the drugs are taken with medications for impotence, such as sildenafil (Revatio, Viagra), vardenafil (Levitra, Staxyn) or tadalafil (Adcirca, Alyq, Cialis).

To reduce your risk of side effects from an alpha-adrenergic blocker, your doctor may start you out with a low dose of the medication and then gradually increase the dosage. If you're already taking medication for high blood pressure, your doctor may monitor you to make sure the alpha blocker doesn't affect your blood pressure.

Topical estrogen

The female bladder and urethra contain receptors for the hormone estrogen, which helps maintain tissue strength and flexibility. After menopause, the female body produces less estrogen. This drop in estrogen is thought to contribute to the deterioration of the supportive tissues around the bladder and urethra, weakening them and increasing the risk of stress incontinence.

Interestingly, oral medications containing estrogen, such as hormone replacement therapy, often worsen urinary incontinence rather than improve it. In addition, oral estrogen is associated with health risks. Therefore, it isn't recommended for treatment of urinary incontinence.

EFFECTIVE BUT TOO DANGEROUS

Drugs such as ephedrine and pseudoephedrine belong to a class of medications called alpha-adrenergic agonists. These drugs and products that contain them can improve symptoms of urge incontinence. But alpha-adrenergic agonists aren't recommended to treat incontinence because of their potential for serious side effects.

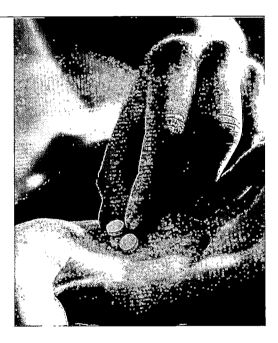

Alpha-adrenergic agonists do the opposite of alpha-adrenergic blockers. Instead of blocking the alpha-adrenergic receptors in the bladder neck and urethra, these drugs stimulate the receptors by mimicking the action of the hormone norepinephrine. The result is contraction of the urethral smooth muscle, tightening the urinary sphincter and preventing urine from leaking out.

The problem is, the medications are also powerful cardiovascular stimulants and can produce dangerous side effects, including severe allergic reactions, chest pain, an irregular heartbeat and difficulty breathing. Other side effects from the drugs include agitation, insomnia, anxiety, dry mouth and headache. Alpha-adrenergic agonists shouldn't be taken if you have glaucoma, diabetes, hyperthyroidism, heart disease or high blood pressure.

Medication	Type of incontinence	Those most likely to benefit
Anticholinergics	Urge incontinence (overactive bladder)	Women and some men
Darifenacin (Enablex)		
Fesoterodine (Toviaz)		
Oxybutynin (Ditropan XL; Gel-nique, Oxytrol as a patch)		
Solifenacin (Vesicare, Vesicare LS)		
Tolterodine (Detrol, Detrol LA)		
Trospium		
Beta-3 adrenergic agonists	Urge incontinence	Men and women
Mirabegron (Myrbetriq)		
Alpha-adrenergic blockers	Urge incontinence	Men
Alfuzosin (Uroxatral)		
Doxazosin (Cardura, Cardura XL)		
Dutasteride (Avodart)		
Dutasteride and tamsulosin (Jalyn)		
Finasteride (Proscar)		
Prazosin (Minipress)		
Silodosin (Rapaflo)		
Tamsulosin (Flomax)		
Terazosin		

Medication	Type of incontinence	Those most likely to benefit
Estrogen	Urge incontinence	Women
Vaginal cream (Estrace, Premarin)		
Vaginal ring (Estring)		
Vaginal tablet (Vagifem)		
Antidepressants	Stress incontinence	Women
Duloxetine (Cymbalta)*		
Imipramine (Tofranil)	Urge incontinence Stress incontinence Mixed incontinence Nighttime incontinence	Men and women
Desmopressin	Bed-wetting	Children
(DDAVP, Nocdurna)	Nighttime incontinence	Some men and women

*Off-label use

Estrogen is also available in the form of a cream, ring or tablet, which may be applied to vaginal areas. Studies have found topical estrogen to be only mildly effective in treating urinary incontinence, and in some cases not much better than an inactive substance (placebo). However, when topical estrogen is used in combination with other treatments, such as pelvic floor muscle training, it may be of some benefit.

Side effects and cautions

Oral estrogen is associated with increased risk of heart disease, stroke, blood clots and breast cancer. Topical estrogen has a much more localized effect than does oral estrogen because not as much of it enters your bloodstream. As a result, it's not likely to produce the overall risks associated with oral hormone therapy.

Antidepressants

Two different types of antidepressant medications are sometimes prescribed.

Duloxetine

Duloxetine (Cymbalta) has been shown in studies to improve symptoms of stress incontinence in women and improve quality of life. Use of this medication to treat urinary incontinence is an unlabeled use, meaning the drug has been approved for other medical conditions, but not specifically for urinary incontinence.

Duloxetine affects the hormones serotonin and norepinephrine, keeping them active for a longer period of time. Some of the effects of this sustained activity are relaxation of the bladder muscle and strengthening of the urethral sphincter, increasing bladder storage capacity while reducing or preventing leakage.

Side effects and cautions

The most common side effect is nausea, but it's usually mild and goes away in a few weeks. Other possible side effects include anxiety, agitation, blurred vision, weight changes and decreased sex drive.

Imipramine

Imipramine (Tofranil) is an older medication and its use is declining. At times, it

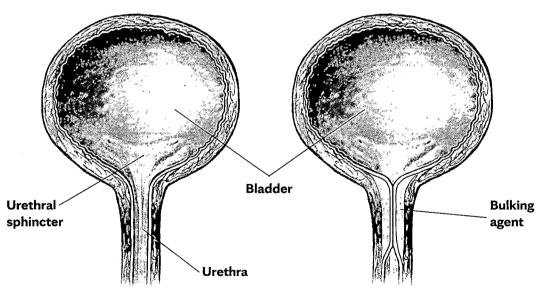

Urethral sphincter   **Bladder**   **Urethra**   **Bulking agent**

Bulking agents are used to help tighten the area where urine flows from the bladder into the urethra. Bulking agents are injected into the tissue near the urethral sphincter to help prevent urine leakage.

may be helpful in the treatment of bladder dysfunction related to a spinal cord injury. It may also be helpful for children who regularly wet the bed at night (nocturnal enuresis).

Side effects and cautions

Imipramine can cause serious side effects involving the cardiovascular system, such as postural hypotension and an irregular heartbeat. Older adults and children may be especially susceptible to these side effects. Other side effects, including dry mouth, blurry vision and constipation, are similar to those of anticholinergics.

Tricyclic antidepressants such as imipramine interact with many different medications, so make sure your doctor knows which medications you're taking before you begin taking this drug.

Desmopressin

Desmopressin (DDAVP, Nocdurna) is a synthetic version of a natural hormone called anti-diuretic hormone (ADH). This hormone slows the production of urine. Your body normally produces more ADH at night, so the need to urinate is lower.

Nighttime bed-wetting (nocturnal enuresis) in children may be caused by a shortage in the nighttime production of ADH. Desmopressin is commonly used to treat nocturnal enuresis in children and is available as a nasal spray or pill for use before bedtime.

A few studies have suggested that desmopressin may also reduce nighttime incontinence in adults. However, the medication is generally less effective in adults than in children.

Side effects and cautions

Side effects are uncommon, but there is a risk of water retention and sodium deficiency in the blood (hyponatremia), particularly in older adults.

INJECTIONS

Urinary incontinence may be treated by injecting substances into tissues and muscles that support the bladder and other urinary organs. These approaches are generally prescribed if medications haven't been successful and surgery isn't an option or isn't preferred.

Bulking agents

Bulking agents are relatively noninvasive, and they may be an option if you would rather try to avoid surgery. Treatment with a bulking agent involves the injection of a material that adds bulk to the tissue surrounding the urethra and the urethral sphincter. This serves to tighten the seal of the sphincter and prevent urine from leaking (see opposite page).

Bulking agents may be particularly useful for women with intrinsic sphincter deficiency (ISD), a condition in which the urethral sphincter muscles don't seal off urine in the bladder, or for men who've had their prostate gland removed. Evidence suggests that bulking agents may also help alleviate stress incontinence due to urethral hypermobility, a condition in which the bladder neck and urethra temporarily shift under pressure.

The bulking agent procedure is done with minimal anesthesia, and it typically takes about five minutes. For most women, the procedure can be done in a doctor's office. For men, the procedure is more involved because of the male anatomy and is more often done in an outpatient sedation area. The standard method of injecting a bulking agent is with a needle, and with the assistance of a cystoscope, a slender, tube-like instrument that allows a surgeon to view the urethral area.

The downside of many bulking agents is that they lose their effectiveness over time, and repeat injections are often needed every six to 18 months.

Following are examples of bulking agents that have been approved by the Food and Drug Administration and are currently in use.

Carbon-coated pyrolytic beads

Carbon-coated pyrolytic beads (Durasphere EXP) have an advantage over some of the other synthetic bulking agents in that the particles are big enough that they won't migrate. Durasphere EXP is nonallergenic, which means it doesn't carry the risk of causing an adverse allergic reaction. A study comparing carbon-coated pyrolytic beads with other bulking agents found them to be equally effective.

Calcium hydroxylapatite particles

Coaptite is the brand name for particles of calcium hydroxylapatite contained within a gel carrier. It's a toothpaste-like substance that's injected into the wall of the urethra near the bladder.

Like other injectable products, it bulks the wall of the urethra to help prevent leakage of urine. A few months after the injection, a part of the gel vanishes but the solid particles remain. Individuals who have received the treatment report a slight to significant improvement in their symptoms.

Silicone

Silicone macroparticles (Macroplastique) are contained in a toothpaste-like gel that's injected into the wall of the urethra near the bladder. After injection, the material bulks the wall of the urethra to help prevent uncontrolled urination. Similar to other bulking agents, repeat injections may be needed.

Bulkamid hydrogel

This recently approved product is a soft, smooth hydrogel that consists mostly of water and a small amount of the polymer polyacrylamide. Once injected, Bulkamid provides additional volume to the urethra and acts as a scaffold for cells to grow around it, helping to provide long-lasting relief of stress urinary incontinence symptoms.

Botulinum toxin type A (Botox)

Among individuals with urge incontinence due to an overactive bladder, behavior therapy and medication are generally the first line of treatment. If these treatments aren't effective or in case of severe symptoms, injections of Botox may be appropriate. Botox may also be injected into the muscles of the bladder to treat incontinence associated with nerve damage. This may include people with a spinal cord injury or Parkinson's disease or children born with spina bifida.

Botox is made from a toxin produced by the bacterium *Clostridium botulinum* that helps stop muscle spasms. When Botox is injected into the bladder muscle, it causes the bladder to relax, increasing the bladder's storage capacity and reducing episodes of urinary incontinence.

The injection is performed with a long, slender instrument that carries a small camera at its tip through which your doctor can view the inside of your bladder (cystoscope). The procedure is often done in an office setting, and is generally effective for six to nine months.

Treatment with Botox can be repeated when the benefits from the previous treatment have decreased, but there should be at least 12 weeks between treatments.

Studies have found that Botox significantly improves symptoms of incontinence and causes few side effects. It reduces the need for medications and catheterization in people with a condition called neuropathic overactive bladder. Botox may also be helpful for some individuals with severe urge incontinence from an overactive bladder that's unrelated to a neurological condition.

The most common adverse reactions observed after injection of Botox into the bladder were urinary tract infection and urinary retention. Individuals who develop urinary retention after Botox treatment may require self-catheterization to empty the bladder.

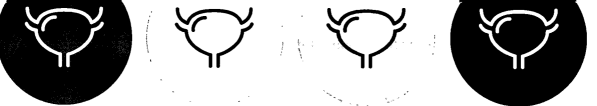
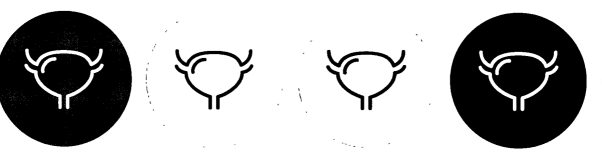
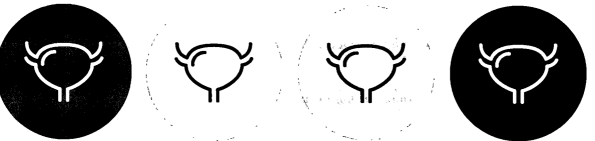
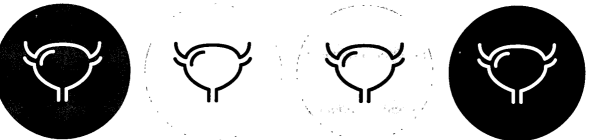
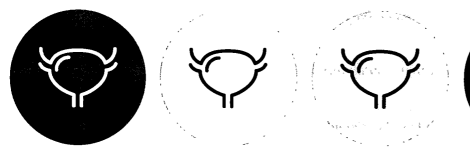
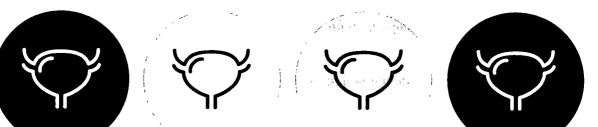

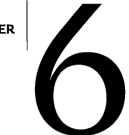

Surgery

In cases where conservative therapies or medications aren't helpful, the next step may be surgery. In general, surgery is reserved for situations in which other types of treatment don't improve symptoms and incontinence is significantly disrupting a person's quality of life.

Surgery is more invasive and has a higher risk of complications than other therapies, but it can also be effective in treating urinary incontinence and provide a long-term solution in severe cases. Most surgical options are used to treat stress incontinence, although surgical alternatives are now available for severe urge incontinence as well.

Before you have surgery to treat your incontinence, it's important to have an accurate diagnosis of your condition

because different types of surgery are used to treat different types of incontinence. Your doctor may refer you to an incontinence specialist (see page 8) for further diagnostic testing and evaluation.

If your incontinence is the result of a separate medical condition, your treatment may be aimed at correcting that condition, which may also resolve your incontinence. For example, if you're a male with overflow incontinence, surgery to treat an enlarged prostate gland that's constricting the urethra and preventing the bladder from emptying may resolve your overflow incontinence.

As with any surgical procedure, surgery for urinary incontinence has the potential for complications such as bleeding, wound infection and organ injury, but these are uncommon. More frequently, urinary tract infection may occur after the operation, particularly if you need to use a catheter for a short period of time. This can be treated with antibiotics.

Although surgery almost always improves urinary incontinence, in some cases it may not completely cure the problem. In addition, surgery can only correct the condition it's designed to treat. If you have mixed incontinence, surgery for stress incontinence won't help urge incontinence. You may need to take medication after surgery to address the urge incontinence. It's also possible that after surgery urinary and genital problems may develop that previously didn't exist, but that's uncommon.

Visiting with your surgeon before having an operation can give you a good idea of the risks and benefits associated with the different types of surgery and help you decide which approach might be best for your particular situation. For example, you may prefer a surgical approach with the lowest risk of complications or the shortest recovery time. Or you may opt for more-extensive surgery that gives you the greatest chance of a complete cure. In addition, your surgeon's experience is likely to play a role in the type of surgery you choose.

Surgery for urinary incontinence is rarely urgent. So, unless your doctor says otherwise, take your time learning about your options and reviewing them with your surgeon. This way, you'll be able to make a decision that's the most likely to leave you satisfied with the results.

WOMEN

Urinary incontinence surgery for women is usually considered only if more-conservative strategies aren't effective. Incontinence surgery is more invasive and has a higher risk of complications than many other forms of treatment, but it can also provide a long-term solution for women with severe cases.

Surgery is most often done to treat severe stress incontinence. However, low-risk surgical alternatives are available for other bladder problems, including severe urge incontinence.

Several procedures have been developed to treat stress incontinence. Most surgical procedures fall into two main categories: sling procedures and bladder neck suspension procedures.

Sling procedures

A sling procedure — the most common surgery to treat stress incontinence — uses a strip of your body's tissue or synthetic mesh material to create a pelvic sling, or hammock, under the bladder neck and the tube that carries urine from the bladder (urethra). The sling provides support to help keep the urethra closed, especially when you cough or sneeze. Slings have been found to be highly effective, and the risk of complications with this type of surgery is low.

Because sling procedures don't require a large abdominal incision, recovery time with this procedure is generally shorter than with more-conventional surgery. Your doctor may recommend two to six weeks of healing before returning to normal activities.

There are three main categories of urethral slings:
- Tension-free
- Adjustable
- Conventional

Discuss with your doctor which type of sling may work best for you based on your medical history and the results of tests to diagnose your condition.

Tension-free slings

Strips of synthetic material or your body's tissues are used to create a tension-free sling. The sling forms a hammock around the urethra and the area of thickened muscle where the bladder connects to the urethra (bladder neck). This helps keep the urethra closed, especially when you cough or sneeze. No stitches are used during surgery to attach the sling. Instead, body tissue initially holds the sling in place. Eventually, scar tissue forms in and around the sling to keep it from moving.

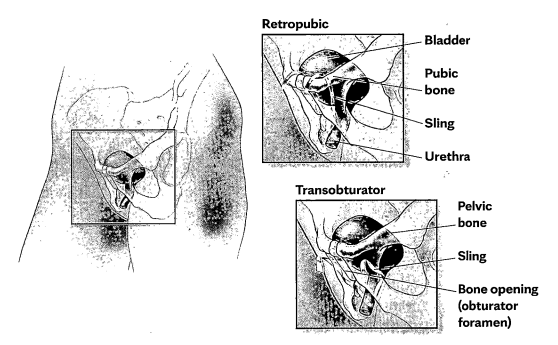

Retropubic
- Bladder
- Pubic bone
- Sling
- Urethra

Transobturator
- Pelvic bone
- Sling
- Bone opening (obturator foramen)

A sling is a piece of tissue or a synthetic material that is surgically placed to support the bladder neck and urethra. Two sling techniques are shown — the retropubic and transobturator. Both are designed to reduce or eliminate stress incontinence in women.

Within the category of tension-free slings, there are three approaches: retropubic, transobturator and single-incision mini.

- **Retropubic.** For the retropubic procedure, a small incision is made inside the vagina just under the urethra, and two small openings are made above the pubic bone. These openings are just large enough for a needle to pass through. To place the sling inside the body, a surgeon uses a needle that's holding the sling. Stitches aren't needed to keep the sling in place, although the vaginal incision is closed with a few absorbable stitches and the needle sites may be sealed with skin glue or sutures.
- **Transobturator.** The transobturator approach is performed slightly differently than the retropubic procedure. It requires a similar vaginal incision, but sling arms aren't passed between the pubic bone and bladder. The needle enters next to the labia and is threaded under the urethra. Like the retropubic approach, stitches aren't needed to hold the sling in place, and the needle site may be sealed with skin glue. The transobturator approach lowers the risk of urethral and bladder injury. However, surgeons generally prefer the retropubic approach because it's more effective.
- **Single-incision mini.** The single-incision minisling utilizes the same concepts of the other tension-free slings, but only one incision is needed to perform the procedure. A small incision is made in the vagina. No incisions are needed in the groin area or the abdomen, and no needles pass through these areas. This decreases the risk of injury. The minisling procedure may be performed in an operating room or under local anesthesia in an outpatient setting or office procedure room. Outcomes with this approach generally aren't as good as with the retropubic and transobturator procedures.

Recovery time with a synthetic mesh sling is fairly short. It's usually only a week or two before you're able to return to your regular activities. Though rare, serious complications from the surgical mesh can occur, including erosion of the material and pain.

Adjustable slings

This type of sling can be adjusted during and after surgery. After the sling is placed and while you're awake, your doctor tests and adjusts the sling's tension according to your needs. Adjustments can continue to be made months or years later and require only a local anesthetic to access the adjustable portion. These types of slings may be used in cases in which a tension-free sling hasn't been effective or in special situations.

Conventional slings

In a conventional sling procedure, a surgeon inserts a sling through a vaginal incision and brings it under the bladder neck. The sling may be made of a synthetic material, your own tissue, animal tissue or tissue from a deceased donor. Using materials taken from animals or deceased donors may be less effective because there's a tendency for the body to absorb animal and deceased donor material.

With a conventional sling, the surgeon brings the ends of the sling through a small abdominal incision and attaches the ends to pelvic tissue (fascia) or to the abdominal wall with stitches to achieve the right amount of tension. This differs from tension-free slings in which tissue friction holds the sling in place instead of stitches.

A conventional sling may require a larger incision and an overnight hospital stay. A temporary catheter may be necessary after surgery as the bladder heals. Conventional slings haven't proved to be better than newer tension-free slings.

Bladder neck suspension procedures

Bladder neck suspension procedures were once the surgery of choice among women with stress incontinence, but

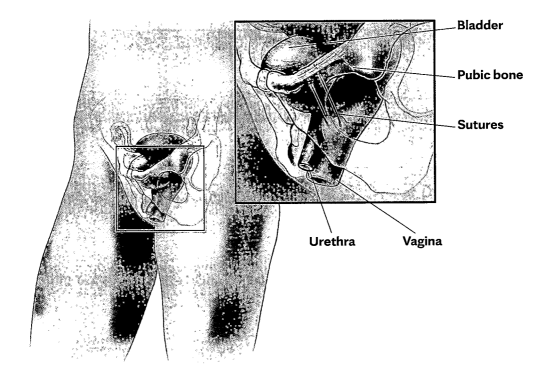

Bladder neck suspension surgery is aimed at adding support to the bladder neck and urethra, reducing stress incontinence. The procedure involves placing sutures in vaginal tissue near where the bladder and urethra meet (bladder neck) and attaching the sutures to ligaments near the pubic bone.

they've become less widely used with the advent of slings. Bladder neck suspension procedures are designed to reduce incontinence by providing added support to the bladder neck and urethra. There are variations of this surgery, and sometimes the procedure may be performed with robotic assistance or laparoscopically, using several smaller incisions instead of one large one.

The most common form of bladder neck suspension surgery is retropubic suspension. For the retropubic suspension procedure, a surgeon places stitches (sutures) in tissue near the bladder neck, bolstering the urethra and bladder neck so that they don't sag.

Retropubic surgery is generally an effective treatment for stress incontinence. The downside of the procedure is that it involves general anesthesia, and recovery can take several weeks, during which time you may need to use a catheter until you can urinate normally. For these reasons, sling procedures are now more commonly used.

Sacral nerve stimulation

For women with severe urge incontinence that can't be controlled with other treatments, sacral nerve stimulation may be an option. In this surgical procedure, a stimulator that looks like a pacemaker is placed under your skin.

Your ability to urinate is governed by a complex set of voluntary and involuntary impulses between your brain and a nerve at the base of your spinal cord, called the sacral nerve, that connects to your bladder. If this communication pathway is disrupted or becomes imbalanced, it can lead to an overactive bladder that sends too many impulses to your brain with the message that you need to urinate. This causes the strong urge to urinate characteristic of urge incontinence.

The purpose of sacral nerve stimulation is to interfere with this imbalance in message transmission by continuously sending small electrical impulses to the sacral nerve. To do this, a surgeon places a thin wire with a small electrode tip near the sacral nerve. The wire is passed under your skin to a small, pacemaker-like device that's placed in a "pocket" of fat beneath the skin of your buttock just below the beltline (see the illustration on the opposite page).

The device contains a battery and electronics that control impulses to the sacral nerve. In addition to controlling a strong urge to urinate, sacral nerve stimulation may also be used to treat urinary frequency and nonobstructive urinary retention.

Because sacral nerve stimulation doesn't work for everyone, your doctor can let you test out the unit first by wearing the pacemaker-like device externally. If the stimulation substantially improves your symptoms, then you can have it implanted in your buttock. Surgery to implant the stimulator is done in an operating room under local anesthesia. Most people are able to go home the same day and recover as an outpatient.

Two types of batteries are used in the stimulation device. Nonrechargeable batteries last for three to five years before they need to be replaced during an outpatient procedure. Rechargeable batteries last for about 15 years. The batteries used in today's devices are also MRI friendly, meaning that you're still able to have a magnetic resonance imaging (MRI) scan if you have a sacral nerve stimulator implanted. Before having an MRI, however, confirm with your doctor that your implant is MRI friendly.

The benefits of sacral nerve stimulation are that it can greatly reduce or eliminate

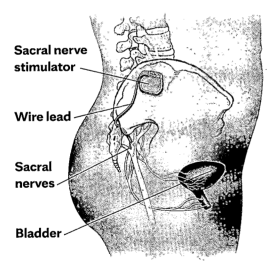

Sacral nerve stimulator

Wire lead

Sacral nerves

Bladder

The sacral nerve stimulator is an electronic device used to stimulate nerves that regulate bladder activity. The unit is placed beneath the skin of the buttocks, about where the back pocket is on a pair of pants. It's shown here out of place for a better view of the unit.

bladder control problems in people who have symptoms of overactive bladder. It's also a type of treatment that can be completely reversed and discontinued at any time without permanent damage to the nerves. In addition, sacral nerve stimulation is an alternative to more-invasive surgery. Risks of complications, including infection, are low. The device can be removed at any time.

Another type of stimulation that's less invasive, called tibial nerve stimulation, is discussed in Chapter 4.

MEN

Similar to surgery for women, urinary incontinence surgery for men is considered only if more-conservative strategies haven't been helpful. Surgery is most often performed to treat overflow incontinence associated with an enlarged prostate gland (benign prostatic hyperplasia, or BPH). For more information on BPH and its treatment, see page 100.

Men with severe urge incontinence that doesn't respond to conservative therapies or medication may be treated with sacral nerve stimulation. For information on this procedure, see the opposite page.

For severe stress incontinence that doesn't improve with conservative measures, there are a couple of options. Researchers are studying the use of an adjustable sling to see if it's as effective in men as it is in women. Another procedure to treat male stress incontinence is placement of an artificial sphincter.

Artificial sphincter

An artificial sphincter is a small device that's particularly helpful for men who have weakened urethral sphincters from treatment of prostate cancer or an enlarged prostate gland. The surgery is rarely used for women unless they have severe incontinence due to intrinsic sphincteric deficiency, and other treatments haven't worked.

Surgery to place the device requires general or spinal anesthesia. The doughnut-shaped device is implanted around the neck of your bladder. Its fluid-filled ring keeps your urethral sphincter closed until you're ready to urinate. To urinate, you press a valve implanted under your skin that causes the ring to deflate and allows urine from your bladder to be released. Once your bladder is empty, the device re-inflates over the next few minutes.

The pump isn't activated until sometime after the surgery so that the area where it was placed has time to heal. For the first four to six weeks after surgery, you'll need to follow a few standard restrictions, such as no driving, no sexual activity, no strenuous activities and no sitting for long periods. In addition, you'll have some permanent restrictions, such as not riding bikes, motorcycles or other vehicles with a similar seat, and not riding horses.

This surgery can cure or greatly improve incontinence in the majority of men with incontinence. A potential disadvantage is that the device may malfunction, requiring additional surgery to fix the problem.

OTHER PROCEDURES

These procedures were once commonly used but now are performed only in rare

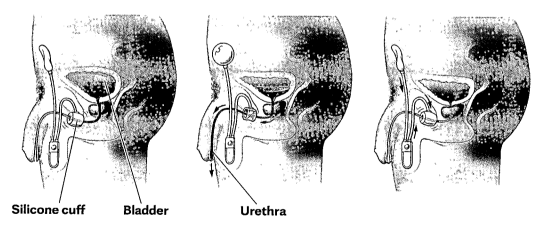

Silicone cuff   **Bladder**   **Urethra**

An artificial sphincter uses a small silicone cuff placed around the urethra to treat incontinence. When inflated, the cuff squeezes the urethra, preventing urine from leaking. To urinate, you deflate the cuff, allowing urine to pass.

circumstances when other treatments aren't effective or possible.

Hydrodistention

Hydrodistention may be used to treat urge incontinence. It's also used to diagnose and temporarily treat inflammation of the bladder wall (interstitial cystitis). The procedure involves filling your bladder with fluid until it's stretched beyond its normal capacity, and keeping it distended for several minutes. Stretching the bladder in this way can be painful, so the procedure is performed under general or local anesthesia.

Doctors aren't exactly sure how hydrodistention works, but the theory is that stretching the bladder wall deadens overly sensitive nerve fibers, reducing the flow of information between the bladder and the brain and decreasing the involuntary contractions characteristic of overactive bladder.

After the procedure, you may experience some pain and discomfort, especially when urinating the first few times. Your urine may contain some blood, but this is normal. Potential complications include bleeding, urinary retention, bladder perforation and interstitial fibrosis, which leads to stiffening of the bladder wall. These are fairly uncommon.

Bladder augmentation

Bladder augmentation is a complex surgery to increase the size of the blad-

der. For a long time, it was the only procedure available for people with debilitating symptoms of urge incontinence. Today, it's rarely performed.

Among some people with urge incontinence, the bladder shrinks over time and empties too frequently. The purpose of bladder augmentation surgery is to increase the size and storage capacity of the bladder by taking a section of small intestine and attaching it to the bladder. The surgery is done under general anesthesia and may take several hours. Many people, especially those with underlying nerve damage, require lifelong use of a catheter after the procedure. Possible side effects of the surgery include infection and chronic diarrhea.

Urinary diversion

Under rare circumstances — such as when an overactive bladder is completely unresponsive to therapy or if all bladder function has been lost — urine may be stored and drained by means other than the bladder and urethra. This is called a urinary diversion.

Your surgeon creates a separate reservoir in your lower abdomen using a segment of your small intestine or colon. He or she then redirects your ureters to the reservoir so that the urine flows into it rather than your bladder. A small opening is made in your abdomen so that the urine can be drained into a bag or through a catheter.

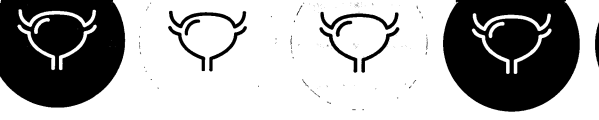
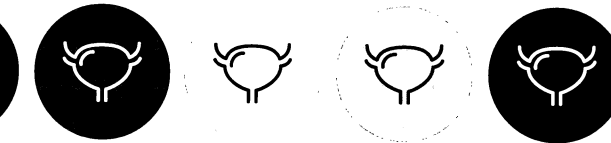
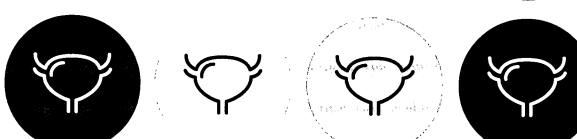
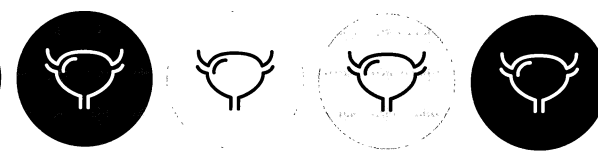
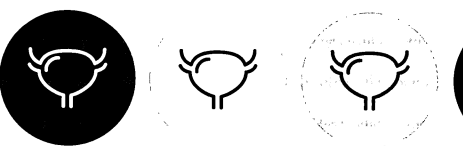
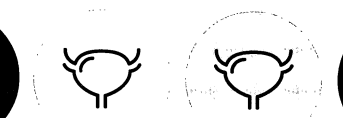

Concerns specific to different groups

7

Although urinary incontinence can affect anyone — men and women, young and old — it's not the same for everyone. Men and women experience it differently, as do children and older adults.

Basic anatomical and hormonal differences account for much of the differentiation between men and women. In women, urinary incontinence commonly results from weakened pelvic floor muscles, which may be caused by various life events and changes such as childbirth and menopause. In men, weakened pelvic floor muscles usually aren't a problem, but issues associated with the prostate gland often contribute to urinary incontinence.

In children, urinary incontinence is frequently transient and gets better with time. In older adults, urinary incontinence often is associated with changes that can occur with aging, the way in which the kidneys and bladder function, and various other factors, as well as diseases that become more common later in life, such as Parkinson's disease and Alzheimer's disease.

Because of these differences, treatment may vary a little or a lot, depending not only on the cause of your incontinence, but also on your sex and your age. This chapter takes a detailed look at urinary incontinence from each of these perspectives.

WOMEN

Urinary incontinence is much more common in women than in men — among individuals younger than age 65, nearly seven times as many women as men experience it. Women may experience all types of urinary incontinence, but stress incontinence is most common.

Urinary incontinence in women often results from wear and tear on the reproductive system as a result of pregnancy and childbirth and hormonal changes associated with menopause. Physical changes resulting from these life events can weaken the pelvic floor muscles and the tissues supporting the urogenital area. Incontinence may also be associated with pelvic organ prolapse, a condition in which one of the pelvic organs, such as the bladder, pushes down on and causes bulging of the vagina. Other less common causes of female incontinence include pelvic surgery and an abnormal connection (fistula) between the vagina and the urethra.

Pregnancy and childbirth

When you're pregnant, particularly during the last trimester, the increasing weight of your uterus places added pressure on the bladder, which can result in stress incontinence. This type of incontinence is usually temporary and goes away after your child is born.

In contrast, the stresses of labor and delivery can have a more lasting effect. Multiple births, prolonged difficult labors, forceps-assisted deliveries and perineal trauma, such as tears or episiotomies, can stretch the pelvic floor muscles and the ring of muscles that surround the

urethra (urinary sphincter). Weakened pelvic floor muscles aren't always able to help keep the bladder neck tightly closed, and this can lead to urine leakage when sudden increased pressure is placed on your bladder. The stress of childbearing also can damage nerves that lead to your bladder, which can also affect your bladder control. Incontinence may develop right after delivery, or it may not occur until many years later.

In most women, it generally takes about three months after delivery for the pelvic floor muscles to regain their natural firmness and elasticity and for incontinence to improve. If you still experience leakage after six months, talk to your doctor about it so that you can be properly diagnosed and decide on a treatment plan. Without treatment, incontinence may become a long-term problem.

Treatment usually includes pelvic floor muscle training (Kegel exercises) with or without biofeedback, and possibly electrical stimulation (see Chapter 4). If your incontinence is severe, you and your doctor may consider surgical options (see Chapter 6). If you're considering having more children, however, you may want to postpone surgery until later. Future pregnancies may cause recurrent incontinence following a successful operation.

You can take steps on your own to help prevent or improve incontinence associated with pregnancy and childbirth by doing Kegel exercises. See page 179 to learn how these are done. Your pelvic floor muscles are just like other muscles in your body. They can be toned and

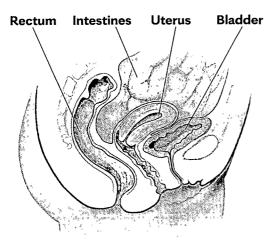

Rectum   Intestines   Uterus   Bladder

Normal anatomy

Pelvic organ prolapse occurs when organs located in your pelvic area — your bladder, uterus, small intestine or rectum — fall or slip out of place (prolapse) and push down on the vagina.

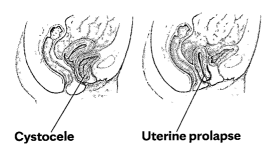

Cystocele   **Uterine prolapse**

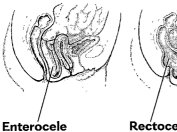

Enterocele   **Rectocele**

firmed with exercise. Doing Kegels regularly throughout your pregnancy and after delivery can strengthen your pelvic floor muscles and improve their effectiveness in keeping your bladder neck closed.

Pelvic organ prolapse

A condition called pelvic organ prolapse — when connective tissue in the pelvis can't support the pelvic organs, causing the organs to fall or slip out of place — may produce both stress and urge incontinence. Often, pelvic organ prolapse produces no symptoms, but in some cases it may produce a feeling of pressure or heaviness or the sense that something is falling out of your vagina. It may even feel like you're sitting on a small ball. Leakage of urine may result, as well as symptoms of frequency and urgency. Difficulty having a bowel movement or discomfort during sex also can occur.

Pelvic organ prolapse occurs because of a lack of pelvic floor muscle support. This can result from childbirth or from estrogen deficiency associated with menopause. Other causes include congenital defects — problems that you were born with, such as absence of a vagina — and pelvic surgery, such as a hysterectomy or even a bladder suspension procedure that was done to treat incontinence. Chronic constipation, heavy lifting and chronic coughing also may contribute to prolapsed pelvic organs.

If you aren't experiencing any symptoms, treatment may not be necessary. However, if the condition is bothersome, your doctor may recommend treatment, beginning with conservative therapies, such as pelvic floor muscle exercises, vaginal estrogen cream or use of a pessary, to provide additional pelvic support. You may also need to avoid heavy lifting and straining.

In cases of severe prolapse, surgery to restore normal positioning of the pro-lapsed organ may be an option. In addi-tion to repositioning the organ, your surgeon may take steps to address incontinence. Chapter 6 has details on surgical procedures to treat incontinence.

Menopause

The hormone estrogen plays a key role in regulating a number of important body functions in women. Among these functions, estrogen helps keep the tissues lining the vagina and urethra healthy and smooth. After menopause the body produces less estrogen. As estrogen levels decline, vaginal and urethral tissues tend to become drier, thinner and less elastic. This affects their ability to close, meaning that part of the protective mechanism that helps maintain continence may be weakened. In addition, age-associated changes unrelated to hormonal changes can lead to a decrease in the bladder's storage capacity.

Some women experience a decline in estrogen production more rapidly than do others. Studies have found that meno-pause in and of itself doesn't represent a strong risk of urinary incontinence. However, when combined with weak

pelvic floor muscle support and tissue damage from childbirth or previous pelvic surgery, vaginal and urethral tissues that are deficient in estrogen can contribute to urinary incontinence.

If you experience urinary incontinence and it seems to be associated with hormonal changes due to menopause, your doctor may recommend estrogen therapy in the form of a vaginal cream, tablet or ring. Although there's no clear evidence that estrogen therapy improves incontinence, it can help tone and revitalize your vaginal and urethral tissues, which may help prevent leakage of urine.

Pelvic surgery

In women, the bladder and uterus lie close to each other and are supported by the same pelvic floor muscles and liga-ments. With any surgery that involves the reproductive system — such as removal of the uterus (hysterectomy) — there's a risk of damage to the muscles or nerves of the urinary tract. This, in turn, can lead to incontinence.

Hysterectomy is one of the most common surgical procedures performed in wom-en, second only to cesarean section. Hysterectomy can be an effective treat-ment for many conditions, including gynecological cancer, uterine fibroids, endometriosis, uterine prolapse and chronic vaginal bleeding.

Although the risk of organ and tissue damage during a hysterectomy is certain-

Certainly not. Not all women who've had children develop incontinence, and in fact, some women who've never had children experience incontinence problems. In addition, hormone fluctuation during menopause isn't as severe in some women as it is in others.

As women become more educated about incontinence, they can take preventive measures early on to exercise and strengthen the muscles that support their reproductive and urinary systems (pelvic floor muscles). This will help reduce the physical stress associated with different life stages and keep these muscles healthy and functional.

---

ly possible, studies of the relationship between hysterectomy and urinary incontinence have been inconclusive. If you're considering a hysterectomy, your doctor can help you assess the risks and benefits in your particular situation.

Urogenital fistula

On rare occasions, an abnormal opening (fistula) between a part of your urinary tract — such as the bladder, urethra or ureter — and your vagina can lead to continuous urinary leakage. Urogenital fistulas may occur after pelvic surgery such as hysterectomy or bladder surgery. The fistula may be caused by injury during surgery, which typically results in immediate leakage.

A fistula may also develop from later complications, such as scar tissue or partial obstruction. In some cases radiation therapy can cause a fistula. In developing countries, urogenital fistulas are more often caused by labor and delivery complications.

If an injury occurs and is noticed while surgery is taking place, your surgeon can repair it immediately. If you develop continuous leakage of urine after surgery and your doctor determines that it's caused by a fistula, additional surgery can be done to repair the opening.

Interstitial cystitis

Interstitial cystitis is a chronic inflammation of the bladder wall. It occurs primarily in women, and its signs and symptoms often resemble those of a urinary tract infection. But unlike a urinary tract infection, urine cultures don't test positive for bacteria.

Signs and symptoms of interstitial cystitis include chronic pelvic pain that may range from a mild burning sensation to severe pain. They also include a frequent

— sometimes urgent — need to urinate, often resulting in urge incontinence. If you have interstitial cystitis, your symptoms may vary over time, periodically flaring in response to common triggers, such as menstruation, sitting for a long time, stress, exercise and sexual activity.

No simple treatment exists to eliminate the signs and symptoms of interstitial cystitis, and no single treatment works for everyone. You may need to try various treatments or combinations of treatments before you and your doctor find the approach that best manages the condition. Treatments include medication, physical therapy and nerve stimulation.

Many people with interstitial cystitis also find that eliminating or reducing their intake of potential bladder irritants (see page 176) helps to relieve their discomfort. Some of the most irritating substances include carbonated beverages, caffeine, and citrus products and food. Artificial sweeteners may aggravate symptoms in some people, as well.

Bladder training techniques (see page 181) may help reduce urinary frequency. Bladder training sometimes involves learning to control the urge to urinate with relaxation techniques. This may include learning to breathe slowly and deeply or learning how to distract yourself with another activity.

MEN

In men, urinary urgency, frequency and incontinence often are related to problems with the prostate gland. The prostate gland, which is about the size and shape of a walnut, is located behind the pubic bone and in front of the rectum. The prostate's main function is to produce most of the fluids in semen, the fluid that transports sperm.

Because of its location, the prostate gland also is important to your urinary health. The gland surrounds the neck of the bladder and upper portion of the urethra much like a doughnut. When your prostate gland is healthy, it doesn't pose any problems. But if disease develops in the prostate, tissue in this gland can swell or grow, squeezing the urethra and affecting your ability to urinate. In addition, urinary incontinence may develop as a complication of surgery to treat prostate problems.

Three types of disease can affect the prostate gland: inflammation (prostatitis), noncancerous enlargement (benign prostatic hyperplasia, or BPH) and cancer. Of these three, BPH is the most common cause of urinary problems, including incontinence. But all three share signs and symptoms of urge and overflow incontinence. Those signs and symptoms include:
- Difficulty starting your urine stream
- A weak urine stream
- The need to urinate more frequently, especially at night
- An urgent need to urinate
- Pain or a burning sensation while urinating
- The feeling that your bladder isn't empty after urinating
- Dribbling of urine after urinating

It's important to note that prostate cancer produces few if any signs and symptoms in its early stages. That's why it's important for men to have regular prostate checkups to identify the disease before it reaches later stages.

Prostatitis

Inflammation of the prostate gland can result from a bacterial infection or another factor that's irritating the gland. Symptoms often include pain or a burning sensation when urinating and trouble urinating. The condition can cause frequent or urgent urination, occasionally resulting in incontinence.

If bacteria are the cause, antibiotics to treat the infection will generally resolve symptoms. Nonbacterial prostatitis, however, is far more common, and it's also more difficult to diagnose and treat because its cause is unknown.

Treatment for nonbacterial prostatitis is often aimed at relieving symptoms. Your doctor may recommend medications to relax the muscles in your bladder neck and urethra and improve urine flow. Pain relievers can help ease pain and discomfort. Other treatment may include biofeedback (see Chapter 4) and exercises to stretch and relax the lower pelvic muscles. Soaking in warm water (a sitz bath) also may help.

NORMAL PROSTATE

ENLARGED PROSTATE

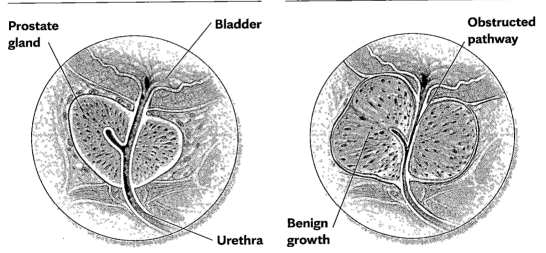

In men, the tube that drains the bladder (urethra), is surrounded by the prostate gland. When tissues in the central portion of the prostate gland enlarge, they can press on the urethra, affecting normal urine flow.

Benign prostatic hyperplasia

At birth, the prostate gland is about the size of a pea. It grows slightly during childhood and then undergoes rapid growth during puberty. By age 25, the prostate is fully developed.

Most men, however, experience a second period of prostate growth in their mid-40s. Frequently at this age, cells in the central portion of the gland — where the prostate surrounds the urethra — begin to expand more rapidly than normal. More than half the men in their 60s and up to 90% of those in their 70s and 80s have some symptoms of benign prostatic hyperplasia (BPH).

As tissues in the center of the prostate enlarge, they often press on the urethra and obstruct urine flow. The bladder needs to work harder to expel urine, and as a result, its wall may become thicker and more irritable. This can lead to increased bladder contractions, even when the bladder contains only small amounts of urine, and increased frequency of urination.

Why the prostate gland enlarges later in life is unclear. Researchers believe that with age the prostate may become more sensitive to the cell growth caused by male hormones such as testosterone. Fortunately, BPH varies in severity and it doesn't always pose a problem. Only about half the men with BPH experience signs and symptoms that are noticeable or bothersome enough to prompt medical treatment. A serious health threat can arise if the condition prevents you from emptying your bladder normally. A bladder that's continually full can lead to recurrent bladder infection and sometimes to kidney damage.

Treatment

Treatment for BPH depends on its severity. If your prostate is enlarged but you're experiencing little or no discomfort, treatment usually isn't necessary. If you have significant problems, a wide variety of treatments are available. In general, treatments aimed at easing signs and symptoms of BPH will also address urinary problems, including incontinence.

Medications are the first line of treatment and the most common method for controlling moderate symptoms of an enlarged prostate. These may include alpha-adrenergic blockers — such as terazosin, doxazosin (Cardura) and tamsulosin (Flomax) — to relax muscles and improve urine flow, or the drugs finasteride (Proscar) and dutasteride (Avodart). Finasteride and dutasteride work by shrinking the prostate gland and are especially helpful for men with large prostates. They're not as effective for men with moderately enlarged or normal-sized prostates or for men with bladders that don't empty completely.

Your doctor may recommend taking a combination of an alpha-adrenergic blocker and finasteride or dutasteride. Researchers have found that combining the two types of drugs can significantly reduce the risk of further prostate gland enlargement to the point where surgery isn't needed. This drug combination also decreases urination problems associated with BPH.

A number of surgical procedures are available for treating BPH. They're mainly for treating severe signs and symptoms, or if you have complications such as frequent urinary tract infections, kidney damage, bleeding through the urethra or bladder stones.

The procedures are often very effective. The most common surgical technique is called transurethral resection of the prostate (TURP), in which a surgeon uses small cutting tools to scrape away excess prostate tissue (see image on page 33). Variations of this procedure also may be performed.

Heat (thermal) therapies are less invasive treatments that use various types of energy — including microwave, radiofrequency and laser — to create heat that destroys excessive prostate tissue. These therapies are generally reserved for small-sized prostate glands. High-energy lasers destroy excess prostate tissue either by vaporizing it or cutting out the tissue.

Treating BPH will generally resolve symptoms of urinary incontinence that often accompany the condition. However, it may take a significant amount of time — six to nine months — for symptoms of incontinence to go away completely. You may need medication to control bladder irritation and incontinence symptoms while you heal from surgery.

Prostate cancer

A cancerous tumor in the prostate gland can press against or block the urethra and cause urination problems, such as overflow incontinence and urinary retention. However, in its early stages, prostate cancer usually doesn't cause any signs or symptoms. And the cancer is often diagnosed before the tumor becomes large enough that it causes a problem. Urinary incontinence is more often associated with the treatment for prostate cancer — surgery or radiation therapy — than the disease itself.

Treatment

Early-stage prostate cancer may be treated with surgery or radiation therapy. Surgical removal of the prostate gland (radical prostatectomy), often performed with robotic assistance, is used to treat prostate cancer that hasn't spread outside of the gland. During the operation, the entire gland is removed as well as surrounding tissues and lymph nodes.

Radiation therapy also can be an effective way to treat prostate cancer. Radiation may be administered two ways: from a machine outside your body (external beam radiation) or through small radioactive seeds implanted in your prostate gland (brachytherapy). Sometimes, both methods are used.

A potential complication of prostate cancer treatment is urinary incontinence. The nerves and muscles that help control urination lie close to the prostate gland,

and depending on the size of the tumor and treatment technique used, it's possible that these nerves and muscles may be damaged during treatment.

Figures vary, but most men have some degree of urinary incontinence after prostate cancer surgery. Among men who receive external beam radiation therapy to treat their cancers, few experience urinary problems. However, symptoms can develop many years after treatment. About one-third of men treated with radioactive seeds develop symptoms of incontinence.

For most men, urinary incontinence after treatment is temporary. Normal bladder control gradually returns over weeks or months as the tissues and nerves heal and strengthen. In some cases, though, incontinence may become chronic. If you experience urinary incontinence after prostate cancer treatment, don't accept it as the price you have to pay for having cancer. In many cases, the problem can be successfully treated.

Stress incontinence that can occur after prostate cancer treatment results from a weakened sphincter muscle. Extra pressure placed on your abdomen during activity can cause urine to leak. To counteract this weakness, your doctor may suggest pelvic floor muscle training (see page 179). Biofeedback or electrical stimulation also may be used to treat stress incontinence. See Chapter 4 for more on these therapies.

Incontinence may also result if during surgery or radiation therapy the nerves that control storage of urine in the bladder are damaged. Incontinence resulting for these reasons requires other types of treatment. The same medications used to treat urge incontinence resulting from an overactive bladder may be prescribed.

CHILDREN

After birth, it generally takes several years for a child to develop the skills needed to remain continent. Initially, a baby's bladder fills to a set point, then contracts and empties automatically. As a child grows, the central nervous system matures and communication between the brain and bladder becomes more defined and efficient. Eventually, a child learns to urinate at will rather than as an involuntary reflex.

Still, accidents can and do happen, particularly at night. This is common, and bladder control often improves with time. In fact, the rate of incontinence in children decreases by approximately 15% for each year after the age of 5. Wetting at night is called nocturnal enuresis. Diurnal incontinence refers to daytime wetting.

Delayed growth is the most common cause for incontinence in children, especially in children who've never been consistently dry. If your child develops incontinence after having been dry for a period of time, it may be due to a recurring urinary tract infection, an overactive bladder, inappropriate urinating habits or a reaction to a stressful life event, such as the birth of a sibling or the first week of school.

Less commonly, incontinence in children may be caused by a neurological condition or anatomical abnormality present at birth (congenital condition).

Nighttime wetting (nocturnal enuresis) is the involuntary urination at night in a child age 5 or older. If your child has never been totally dry, this is known as primary enuresis. If your child was fully trained and then starts bed-wetting after a period of being completely dry, this is referred to as secondary enuresis.

Primary enuresis

Experts don't know the exact cause of primary enuresis, but it most likely arises from a mix of factors that include the following:

Small bladder capacity

Your child's bladder may not be developed enough yet to hold urine through the night.

Excessive nighttime urine production

Up to adolescence, your child's body produces increased levels of anti-diuretic hormone at night. This causes urine production to slow and allows your child to sleep through the night without being bothered by a full bladder. If your child's body isn't producing enough anti-diuretic hormone at night, his or her bladder may fill to the point of overflowing.

Overactive bladder at night

Some children experience uninhibited bladder contractions at night, leading to bed-wetting. An overactive bladder at night usually is connected to daytime symptoms such as frequency, urgency and "holding on," and to low bladder capacity. If your child is having both daytime and nighttime signs and symptoms, he or she has functional incontinence. This is generally treated differently from nocturnal enuresis.

Trouble waking up or leaving bed

Whether your child has a small bladder, excessive nighttime production of urine or an overactive bladder, the bed-wetting occurs because of an inability to wake up to go to the toilet or difficulties reaching the toilet. Although children who wet the bed sleep normally — that is, they don't necessarily sleep any more deeply than other children — they're unable to rouse themselves when their bladders are full.

Studies show that bed-wetting typically occurs in the first third of the night, which also happens to be when it's most difficult for all children to wake up. In some cases, a child may wake up but may not want to get out of bed for fear of the dark or because it's cold. In these situations, practical measures such as leaving a hall light on or keeping the room warm may help.

Genetics

Bed-wetting appears to run in families. If both parents experienced nocturnal enuresis as children, the chance of their children experiencing it is increased.

Primary enuresis treatment

When deciding on a treatment plan for your child, it's important to include your child in the discussion. Evidence indicates that when a child understands the emotional as well as the practical benefits of being dry and is motivated to stop wetting, treatment is generally more successful. In some cases, formal treatment may not even be necessary. The child may become dry without any further treatment.

Key ingredients to a positive treatment plan include:
- Instituting regular patterns of sleeping, eating and drinking throughout the day, as well as regular voiding
- Limiting fluids before bedtime
- Keeping bedtime routines relaxed
- Understanding that the condition is common, it isn't usually a sign of a psychological problem and it often stops on its own

Additional methods for treating nocturnal enuresis include enuresis alarms, behavior therapy and medications. In general, researchers have found the alarm to be the most successful treatment for enuresis, although it's often combined with various behavior modification techniques or medications.

Enuresis alarm

An enuresis alarm is a device that attaches to your child's pajamas. When the device's pad starts to get wet, the alarm goes off, waking up your child. Upon waking, pelvic floor muscles tighten and stop the flow of urine, allowing your child to make his or her way to the toilet to finish urinating.

The purpose of the alarm is to allow your child to learn to respond to the sensation of a full bladder. Alarms usually work best for children older than age 7 who can eventually take some responsibility for waking and going to the toilet on their own. It generally takes about six to eight weeks for this type of therapy to be effective.

Behavior therapy

Behavior modification techniques may be helpful in encouraging your child to develop habits and behaviors that contribute to dryness, such as using the toilet regularly during the day, urinating before going to bed, or waking up to go to the toilet. You may want to create a reward system, such as tokens for favorite activities, to encourage progress and cooperation with bedtime routines.

Because bed-wetting itself is involuntary, avoid punishment and be sure to reward only those behaviors that are under your child's control. Other behavior techniques include scheduled toilet trips throughout the night that are gradually decreased as dryness increases.

Medications

Your doctor may recommend a medication called desmopressin (DDAVP) to increase anti-diuretic hormone levels at night and reduce urine production.

Imipramine (Tofranil) is an antidepressant that may be used to treat nocturnal enuresis and is approved for use in children. For more information on these medications, see Chapter 5. Medications can provide short-term relief of symptoms, but they usually don't offer a cure.

Secondary enuresis

Secondary enuresis may develop temporarily as a result of anxiety due to stressful events, such as a family illness or separation from a parent. Tension in the family or negative attitudes regarding the wetting can exacerbate this anxiety, leading to more wetting and creating a cycle of wetting and anxiety. Behavior factors that may contribute to enuresis include difficulties in sleeping, eating or drinking patterns, lack of cooperation with parents, or self-esteem issues.

Some researchers argue that the speed at which a child first became dry influences his or her susceptibility to secondary enuresis when stress or a crisis arises.

If your child develops secondary enuresis, have him or her examined by a doctor to rule out any underlying physical problems, such as a urinary tract infection, seizure disorder or diabetes. If the problem appears to be a reaction to

stress, your child may benefit from psychotherapy or family therapy.

Daytime wetting

Daytime urinary incontinence is less common than nighttime incontinence but it's similar in that it often goes away on its own. If your child has more than the occasional accident during the day, a visit to your doctor is a good idea to find out what may be causing the incontinence. Daytime incontinence is generally divided into categories.

Overactive bladder

As in adults, overactive bladder in children is characterized by an urgent need to urinate. Children, however, tend to counter this urge by voluntarily contracting their pelvic muscles in order to postpone a trip to the bathroom and minimize leakage. Signs and symptoms may become worse toward the end of the day, as fatigue and loss of concentration increases.

Delaying urination for extended periods of time can increase the risk of a urinary tract infection. In turn, an infection can irritate the bladder and produce further symptoms of urgency and frequency. Damp clothing is also ideal for bacterial growth, which can lead to more infection. All of these factors combined can create a cycle of incontinence and recurrent infection that can sometimes be difficult to treat. Postponing trips to the bathroom to urinate can also lead to postponement of defecation, resulting in constipation and sometimes fecal incontinence.

Treatment for overactive bladder may include anticholinergic medications to decrease involuntary bladder muscle contractions, reduce the strength of the contractions and increase bladder storage capacity. Medical care may also include bladder training and treatment of associated urinary tract infections and constipation. For more on anticholinergic medications, see Chapter 5.

Abnormal urinating habits

Some children will urinate only long enough to reduce the urge, leaving the toilet without completely emptying the bladder, a practice called interrupted voiding. In other children, urine flow is characterized by periodic bursts of pelvic floor contractions so that the flow takes on a staccato pattern. In both conditions, the child is unable to completely relax the pelvic floor muscles. This may occur as a result of constantly trying to counter the urge to urinate, or it may be a learned behavior. These abnormal urinary habits (dysfunctional voiding) can result in urine being left in the bladder, which increases the risk of a urinary tract infection.

Constipation also may be associated with dysfunctional voiding. If stool fills up the rectum and colon, it can put pressure on, or even obstruct, the bladder so that it cannot empty completely. Urine left in the bladder may lead to growth of bacteria and infection. Pressure on the bladder

can irritate the bladder and cause it to contract. These contractions can lead to wetting accidents.

The goal of treatment is to relax the pelvic floor muscles to achieve normal urine flow and completely empty the bladder. This can be done through timed voiding and behavioral training, encouraging children to relax their pelvic muscles when going to the bathroom and taking their time to make sure the bladder is fully emptied. If overactive bladder is present, anticholinergic medications may be added. In the case of constipation, it can often be treated with diet and behavior changes.

Lazy bladder syndrome

Lazy bladder syndrome is the opposite of an overactive bladder. Instead of symptoms of urgency and frequency, children with lazy bladder syndrome feel little or no urge to urinate. When they do go to the bathroom, they must strain their abdominal muscles to expel urine because the bladder fails to contract normally.

Treatment for lazy bladder syndrome consists of using clean, intermittent catheterization to empty the bladder, combined with treatment for infections and constipation.

Giggle incontinence

Some children experience urine leakage when they laugh. Exactly why this happens isn't known. The condition can affect boys and girls and it can last into the teenage and, occasionally, adult years. In general, however, this type of incontinence goes away on its own. The drug methylphenidate has proved effective in treating giggle incontinence in some children.

Neurogenic bladder and anatomical abnormalities

Incontinence caused by a nerve-damaging disease is often referred to as neurogenic bladder. In children, the most common cause of neurogenic bladder is spina bifida. Babies born with spina bifida typically have an outpouching of membranes covering the spinal cord (myelomeningocele) that causes the loss of neurological control of the legs, bladder or bowel.

Surgery is performed soon after birth to minimize the risk of infection and preserve existing function of the spinal cord. Increasingly, spina bifida is being diagnosed and even treated before the baby is born (prenatally). Children with cerebral palsy also may experience incontinence, but this is more often due to lack of mobility than nerve injury.

Treatment for incontinence due to a neurogenic bladder primarily consists of intermittent catheterization and medication. Together, these treatment methods often can achieve dryness in the vast majority of children with this condition. In some cases, surgery may be needed to help achieve dryness.

Rare anatomical abnormalities such as defects of the urethra or ureters also may cause incontinence. These abnormalities can generally be corrected with surgery.

OLDER ADULTS

As you age, a number of changes take place in your body that can make incontinence more likely to occur. These changes include:
- Decreased bladder capacity
- Less elastic bladder walls
- Increased urine retention after urination
- Weakened pelvic floor muscles, particularly in women
- Increasingly overactive bladder
- Enlarged prostate in men

Now, just because these changes take place doesn't mean incontinence will occur. Some older adults experience all of these changes and don't have any bladder leakage problems. Aging is not a direct cause of incontinence. Rather, it increases the risk of incontinence. This is important to note because many older people feel that incontinence is inevitable and that there's nothing that can be done about it. This isn't true. Treatment for incontinence is often effective, in young and old alike.

Urge incontinence from an overactive bladder is the most common type of incontinence in older adults. In addition, many people experience frequent urges to urinate but have weak bladder contractions (detrusor hyperactivity with impaired contractility), which makes it difficult to empty the bladder completely. This can lead to urine retention and, in severe cases, overflow incontinence. Stress incontinence is common among older women. Mixed incontinence also is common among older women and may involve stress incontinence and overactive bladder.

The primary difference in incontinence between younger individuals and older adults is that in older adults, a number of other conditions may be present that increase the risk of incontinence. Some of these are reversible, such as infection, and some are not, such as dementia.

If you're an older adult with incontinence, you and your doctor will need to take into account additional factors that could be related to the development of your incontinence, in addition to actual urinary tract problems. These include mental status, mobility, manual dexterity, motivation and medical issues including bowel habits.

Addressing some of these other risk factors may help to manage or alleviate the incontinence. In fact, in some people, early management of certain risk factors can even prevent incontinence from developing.

Assessment and evaluation

A thorough assessment and evaluation is essential to diagnosing anyone with incontinence. But because so many different factors may contribute to incontinence in older adults — including

factors not directly related to the lower urinary tract — a complete physical examination and continence assessment are typically done, in addition to consideration of the following areas:
- Thinking and judgment skills (cognitive abilities)
- Ability to move around
- Environment, including access to a toilet
- Degree of independence in terms of daily living activities
- Level of support or care
- Potentially reversible contributors to incontinence
- Medications being taken that may lead to or worsen incontinence

Treatment

Age, frailty or disability should not keep a person from receiving treatment for incontinence. In general, older adults are eligible for the same treatment that's available for younger people, with a few caveats.

Behavior therapy

Pelvic floor muscle training, biofeedback, electrical stimulation and bladder training can be effective forms of therapy for older adults who are fit, alert and motivated to take part in their own treatment. For those who have a disability, are frail or have a cognitive impairment, assisted voiding or prompted voiding — where a caregiver periodically reminds the person to urinate — can help prevent accidents and manage incontinence. For more on behavior therapy, see Chapter 4.

NOCTURIA

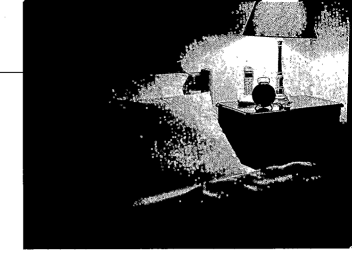

With age, many adults find they need to get up during the night to go to the bathroom (nocturia). Although most people find it acceptable to get up once during the night to urinate, having to get up multiple times can lead to disrupted sleep, drowsiness during the day and an increased risk of falling. In some cases, nocturia can result in incontinence and bed-wetting.

The main causes of nocturia are a decrease in the bladder's ability to hold urine, overproduction of urine or a combination of the two. A smaller bladder volume generally results from aging. Increased production of urine may result from medical conditions, such as diabetes, congestive heart failure or kidney disease. In addition, drinking too much fluid later in the day, long-term use of water pills (diuretics), or changes in posture from day to night that can lead to the transfer of fluid from swollen feet or hands to the kidneys and subsequently to the bladder also may increase urine output. Reduced production of anti-diuretic hormone at night also can lead to increased urine production.

Some people mistake insomnia or waking from sleep apnea or snoring as a need to go to the bathroom. Treating the sleep disorder often addresses the nocturia.

Simple measures may help relieve symptoms of nocturia, including the following:
- Drinking most of your fluids in the morning and early afternoon and limiting how much fluid you drink, particularly alcohol and caffeine, in the late afternoon and evening
- Wearing compression stockings to reduce swelling in your legs and feet
- Elevating your feet in the early evening to reduce swelling and encourage urination before you go to bed
- Changing the time you take your medications

If these efforts don't work, your doctor may prescribe a diuretic that you take late in the afternoon to eliminate fluid retention.

Medications

Incontinence medications are generally prescribed with caution in older adults because of a greater potential for side effects. Still, anticholinergic medications can improve the effectiveness of behavior therapy for urge incontinence, and they may be used in conjunction with bladder training or prompted voiding. In men with enlarged prostates, alpha-adrenergic blockers may be precribed to help empty the bladder.

Before medication is prescribed, it's a good idea to talk with your doctor or other medical provider about all the other medications you're taking to make sure they're not directly or indirectly contributing to your problem. If so, your provider may be able to adjust them to decrease the risk of incontinence. New medications are usually started at a low dose and gradually increased, as needed, to relieve symptoms and minimize side effects.

Medications may sometimes have undesired effects. For example, many people with detrusor hyperactivity with impaired contractility have an overactive bladder but also experience signs and symptoms of urine retention, which can lead to overflow incontinence. Anti-cholinergics may help relax an overactive bladder muscle but may cause incomplete emptying of the bladder and urine retention, worsening overflow incontinence.

Because medications can produce mixed results, they're typically reserved as a secondary form of treatment, usually in combination with behavior therapy.

Surgery

A person's age in and of itself isn't a reason to avoid surgery. Healthy older adults generally respond well to surgery for incontinence and generally can be treated in the same way as younger adults. However, in any older adult who has surgery, there's a risk of postoperative complications, including dehydration, infection, delirium and falls.

Because of the complex nature of incontinence in older adults and the increased risks associated with surgery, doctors typically do a careful evaluation of the problem, including urodynamic testing, to make sure there aren't treatments other than surgery that can address the incontinence. It may be worthwhile to try out conservative treatments first and then reevaluate your condition before having surgery. For more on surgery to treat incontinence, see Chapter 6.

Seek help

If you're an older adult and are experiencing incontinence or you're caring for an older adult with incontinence, seek help for this condition as soon as you can. Your doctor can help you find appropriate treatment and help you sort through the various factors that may be contributing to the problem. Addressing these issues can improve bladder control as well as the quality of life of both the person with incontinence and the caregiver. Bladder control is important to every person's well-being and dignity and is a worthwhile goal.

Diseases that damage the nervous system, such as multiple sclerosis, Parkinson's disease and stroke, can have an effect on bladder control and lead to incontinence. Diseases that cause dementia, such as Alzheimer's, may lead to incontinence due to impaired functioning.

In the beginning stages of a chronic disease, many people can care for themselves with a limited amount of help. But as the disease progresses, a caregiver becomes necessary to assist with the activities of daily living. For someone who's had a stroke, caregiving may be needed immediately after the event. Caring for someone who has incontinence due to a neurological condition is a challenging task, and it often requires a creative approach.

Here are some suggestions that may help:
- Be sure to have the incontinence evaluated by a doctor. It may be due to a reversible condition, such as an infection or a medication. Treating the underlying problem in this case usually improves the incontinence.
- Provide frequent reminders to use the toilet. Generally, a pattern of going to the bathroom every one to two hours works well. You may need to bring the person to the bathroom and provide help with clothing and seating.
- Watch for nonverbal signs, such as pacing or other signs of agitation, that indicate the person needs to use the toilet. He or she may not recognize the feeling of a full bladder or may lack the verbal skills to state this need.
- Avoid clothing with complicated fasteners, such as button-fly jeans. Elastic waistbands work well.
- Leave the door to the bathroom open and a light on to help the person easily locate the room, particularly at night. Some caregivers put reflective tape on the floor in the shape of arrows that point to the location of the bathroom.
- For an individual with dementia, put a picture of a toilet and a sign that reads "Toilet" on the bathroom door. Avoid the words "restroom" or "bathroom," which may be taken literally.
- Dehydration is fairly common in older adults. Don't decrease fluids unless the person is drinking more than eight to 10 glasses a day. Withholding fluids may actually increase incontinence by making urine more concentrated, which can irritate the bladder and cause increased frequency and urgency. However, you may want to discourage more than one beverage after dinner to decrease the occurrence of nighttime incontinence.

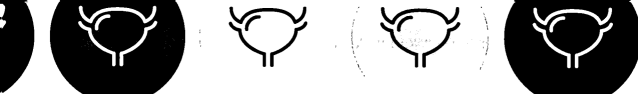
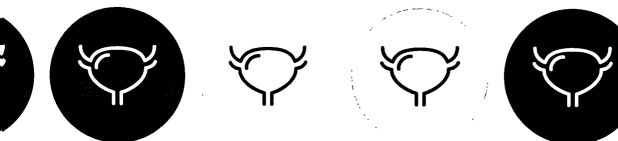
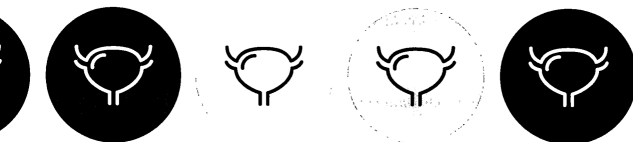
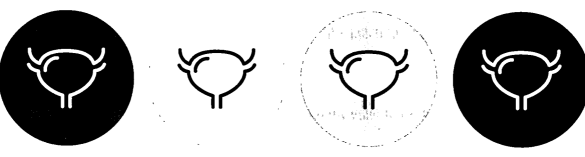
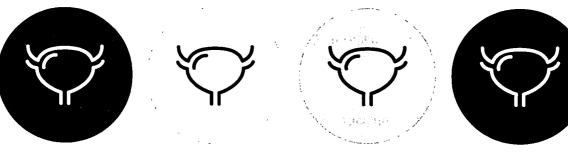
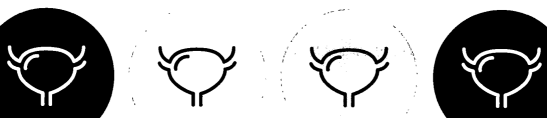

Living well with incontinence

8

The good news about urinary incontinence is that treatment for this condition is becoming more effective. For years, people have managed their incontinence with absorbent pads, by carrying an extra set of clothes, or by simply opting out of social settings and staying at home. Although these methods may help you avoid embarrassment, they don't address the problem.

Today there are better ways to manage urinary incontinence. Behavior therapies, medications, and surgical procedures can substantially reduce, if not eliminate, urinary leakage and help you regain bladder control. In addition, new treatments are continually being discovered. This is why it's important to talk with a specialist who's prepared to help you find the best treatment for your situation. If

you can find a treatment that works — and most people do — you'll greatly minimize the effect of incontinence on your life.

You may still need to cope with the effects of incontinence while waiting to have surgery or for medications or behavior therapies to become effective. And in some instances, treatment may not provide a complete cure. During these times, practical strategies to deal with incontinence — such as reducing risks and modifying your environment — may help.

REDUCING YOUR RISK

Clearly, some risk factors for incontinence are outside of your control, such as aging or a spinal cord injury. But you do have control over other factors, such as lifestyle habits. Eating well, exercising regularly and not smoking are basic components of a healthy lifestyle. Taking steps to improve your lifestyle may reduce your risk of urine leakage and many other health conditions.

Eat and drink well

What goes into your body has a definite effect on your health. Choosing healthy foods and beverages that nourish and strengthen your bones, muscles, organs, and other tissues is vital to helping you feel your best and reducing your risk of illness. The following steps may be particularly helpful for incontinence.

Add fiber to your diet

Constipation is an important contributor to incontinence. Keeping your bowel movements soft and regular allows urine to flow freely, and it reduces the strain that's placed on your pelvic floor muscles. Eating foods that are high in fiber — whole grains, legumes, fruits and vegetables — can help to relieve and prevent constipation. Plus, high-fiber foods are healthy!

Avoid bladder irritants

Avoiding or reducing food and beverages that you know irritate your bladder can help relieve some symptoms of incontinence. For example, if you know that

drinking coffee throughout the day has a tendency to make you go to the bathroom more frequently, you might limit your caffeine intake to one or two cups a day. For a list of potential dietary bladder irritants, see page 176.

Maintain proper fluid intake

Drinking too much fluid can make you urinate more frequently. But not drinking enough can lead to a concentration of waste in your urine, which can irritate your bladder and cause symptoms of urgency and frequency. The daily fluid recommendation for adults is about 60 ounces, approximately eight 8-ounce glasses. But not everyone needs that much. Remember that it doesn't have to be just water. You can get fluids from tea, juice, and foods such as fruits, vegetables and soups.

Lose weight

If you're overweight, losing excess pounds can help reduce overall pressure on your bladder, pelvic floor muscles and associated nerves. Studies suggest that losing just 5% to 10% of your body weight may improve symptoms of incontinence.

There are many ways to lose weight. Crash diets are usually the least effective in the long term. A more effective way is to develop better eating habits and pay attention to the amounts of calories and fat you consume each day. You want to eat foods that are low in energy density. Energy density is a ratio of calories to the volume of food. Fruits and vegetables have low energy density. You can eat large amounts of them and still consume fewer calories than if you eat a small amount of a rich dessert or fried food, which has a lot of calories per volume.

By replacing calorie-dense foods with foods that contain fewer calories per volume, you'll satisfy those hunger pangs while consuming fewer calories. A good way to begin is simply to eat more fruits and vegetables each day and fewer processed and high-fat foods.

Exercise

Getting 30 minutes or more of physical activity most days of the week can improve your fitness and your health. Regular physical activity has many benefits.

- *Strengthens your muscles.* Exercise preserves bone mass and muscle tone. Staying physically active helps keep your muscles — including your pelvic floor muscles — strong and flexible.
- *Reduces weight.* If you're overweight and you need to lose weight, regular exercise can help you shed pounds. A healthy diet and daily exercise is the best approach to losing weight and keeping it off.
- *Prevents prostate enlargement.* In men, walking a total of two or three hours a week can reduce the risk of developing an enlarged prostate gland. Prostate enlargement is one of the most common causes of male incontinence.
- *Preserves independence.* For older adults, regular exercise helps maintain

independence. Exercise can reduce the risk of incontinence caused by restricted mobility or difficulty in managing zippers and buttons. Strengthening your muscles and bones also can improve your balance and coordination, reducing your risk of falls.
- *Fights depression.* Physical activity helps combat depression, which may be associated with incontinence, especially in middle-aged women. Exercise fights depression by helping to balance brain chemicals that may be out of sync. Exercise also stimulates the production of endorphins — brain chemicals that produce feelings of well-being.

Women who experience urine leakage while exercising may consider wearing a device such as a urethral or vaginal insert, which helps prevent leakage. Some women use super tampons or a diaphragm for support. For more on supportive devices, see Chapter 4.

Don't smoke

Smoking can produce a severe chronic cough, which can aggravate symptoms of stress incontinence. Stopping smoking can relieve your coughing, reducing the pressure that coughing places on your bladder and pelvic floor muscles. Plus, stopping smoking has many other benefits, including lowered risk of lung cancer, cardiovascular disease and infertility.

Giving up tobacco is often easier said than done, but it's not impossible. Doing so often involves the use of several

SELF-CARE PRODUCTS FOR INCONTINENCE

A wide variety of products are available. Which ones you choose depends on the volume of urine you tend to lose, when you typically experience leakage, how easy a product is to use, and its cost, comfort, odor control and durability. Your medical provider can help you choose products that will help you the most. You can find incontinence care products at drugstores or medical supply stores and through companies that sell durable medical equipment.

Bladder control pads

Disposable pads designed to manage urine leakage are similar to sanitary pads but are much more absorbent, and they have a waterproof backing. The pads are worn inside your underwear or briefs and discarded after use. Absorbent products generally incorporate three layers: a top layer that wicks away moisture from your skin, a middle layer that absorbs the moisture, and an outer layer that may be waterproof to keep the moisture in or breathable to allow the moisture to evaporate. Sanitary pads may work for very small amounts of leakage, but they generally aren't as absorbent as incontinence pads.

Protective undergarments and products

These products are worn in place of your normal underwear. They include:

- *Pull-ons* Pull-ons function as their name suggests. You pull them up over your legs and wear them like traditional underwear. They're available in either disposable or reusable forms. The disposable forms come in a variety of sizes and absorbencies. The reusable undergarments are washable and come in a couple of varieties. One is made of waterproof material and is designed to be worn as an extra layer of protection over absorbent pads or undergarments. The other kind is newer and is designed to absorb and protect just like a disposable, but it can be washed and reused.
- *Adult briefs* They attach around your waist with either refastenable tape tabs or reusable belts. They're useful for containing large amounts of urine. Some are designed especially for overnight use. Adult briefs are available in both disposable and reusable forms, and they come in a variety of sizes. Some are contoured to better fit the outline of your body.
- *Skin care and odor products* Cleansing wipes and cleansing sprays or foams are gentler to your skin than is toilet paper, and they moisturize your skin and help eliminate odor. Baby wipes work well, too. Special creams, gels or ointments are available that can be used to create a moisture barrier and keep your skin dry. Some ointments also heal irritated skin while acting as a moisture barrier. A pharmacist or your doctor can provide more information.

strategies, including medications and regular visits with a medical provider for counseling and support. Smoking cessation programs also offer supportive guidance on how to stop.

MODIFYING YOUR ENVIRONMENT

If you have trouble getting to the bathroom on time because of restricted mobility, perhaps because of arthritis or recent hip surgery, making a few changes within your home may help you prevent incontinence episodes. Some changes that may be helpful include the following:

- Having your bedroom or sleeping area close to the bathroom
- Keeping the path to the bathroom well-lit and free of obstacles that may get in your way or cause you to trip and fall
- Installing an elevated toilet so that it's easier to sit down and get up
- Installing grab bars to help you get on and off the toilet
- Keeping a bedpan or urinal in your bedroom
- Having a commode (portable toilet) nearby if your only bathroom is up or down a flight of stairs

If you need more-extensive changes, you might consider adding another bathroom to your house in a more convenient location or widening an existing bathroom doorway.

Consulting with an occupational therapist also may be helpful. Occupational therapists specialize in helping people deal with the effects of aging, illness or injury in the management of their daily lives. An occupational therapist can meet with you on an individual basis and make recommendations based on your individual needs.

For example, if you have arthritis and it's difficult for you to maneuver zippers or buttons, an occupational therapist can provide you with tools and tips to make unzipping or unbuttoning your pants easier.

Proper clothing

If you have an overactive bladder and you go to the bathroom frequently, it may help if you limit the number of articles of clothing you wear. Dressing in a number of layers can make it difficult to get to the toilet in time.

For example, women may choose to wear dresses without nylons instead of pants. Men may choose to wear suspenders or pants with an elastic waistband instead of a belt. This way you won't be fumbling with your clothing as your sense of urgency increases. As you gain more control of your bladder through training or timed voiding, you can feel more comfortable wearing different items of clothing.

GETTING OUT AND ABOUT

Try not to let your bladder problems keep you away from work or social settings outside of your home. In fact, it's essential that you maintain your connection with family, friends and colleagues because

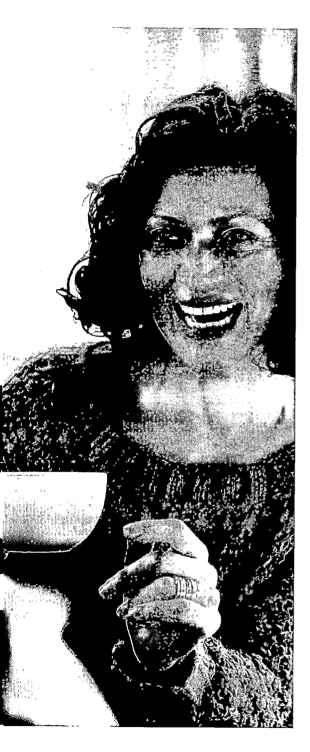

this type of support network can prevent feelings of isolation and depression that can accompany incontinence. Getting out of the house for lunch with a friend or for a movie with your spouse can refresh your perspective and give your spirits a boost.

Behavior therapies such as pelvic floor muscle training and bladder training can help you gain better control over your bladder so that you can last through a meeting at work or a movie at the theater without having to go to the restroom. In the meantime, being prepared can make you feel more confident when you're out and about. The following tips may be helpful. But remember, these are short-term methods for relieving the symptoms of incontinence. They aren't considered a primary form of treatment.

Carry supplies

When going out, take an adequate supply of incontinence pads or protective undergarments with you. This way, if an accident does occur, you can feel confident knowing that you can replace a used product with a fresh one and not have to go home immediately. Today's products are becoming ever more discreet and can easily fit into a roomy purse or small backpack.

You may also wish to carry a change of clothes with you. Even a sweater wrapped around your waist can come in handy in case of an emergency. Carry a zippered plastic bag to place soiled clothing in until you get home.

People who travel a lot often keep a bag of toiletries handy, so they don't need to repack it every time they leave. You could do the same, keeping a bag with all of your necessary supplies by the door, so you can simply grab it on your way out. You might even keep some extra supplies in your car in case you forget your bag.

If an accident does occur, remember that if it's addressed promptly, odor and skin irritation are rarely more than a momentary problem. It's important, though, to take good care of your skin and keep it as dry as possible. Prolonged contact with wet clothing can cause the skin to break down, resulting in irritation and sores.

Scout out your destination

Familiarize yourself with the restrooms available at the place you're going to. If you're at a movie theater or a religious service, you may wish to sit near the aisle so that you can easily get up and go to the restroom if necessary.

If you're accompanying an older adult who has a problem with incontinence, you might go to the restroom yourself every couple of hours and offer him or her the opportunity to go with you. This saves the person the embarrassment of having to ask or be asked to use the restroom.

SEXUALITY AND INCONTINENCE

Sexuality and incontinence are topics that many people find difficult to talk

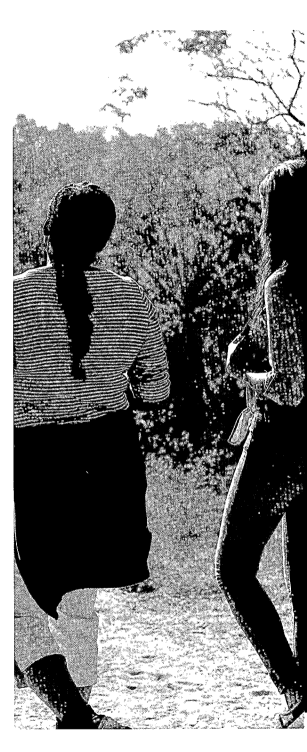

about, and combining the two into one conversation can be even more intimidating. Certainly, incontinence can have a negative effect on your sex life if you let it. But it doesn't necessarily have to get in the way of intimacy.

Leaking urine during sexual intercourse can be upsetting. Women with stress incontinence may find that they leak urine at the beginning of intercourse when their partner's penis presses against the urethra and bladder upon initial penetration. In women with urge incontinence, urine leakage may be more unpredictable, though it often occurs during orgasm, and in greater volume than in women with stress incontinence. The worry that this could happen may prevent you from feeling relaxed during a sexual experience.

Pelvic organ prolapse in women is another reason for sexual inactivity. Other factors associated with the problem include emotions, experiences, beliefs, lifestyle and your relationship with your partner.

Men who have incontinence associated with prostate cancer treatment also may have erectile dysfunction, a common side effect of prostate surgery. In this case, erectile dysfunction is likely to be a greater factor in sexual discomfort than is incontinence. Men don't usually leak urine during intercourse because of penile engorgement.

If you feel that problems with incontinence are affecting your sex life or your sexuality in general — how you feel about yourself as a sexual being — consider having a frank discussion with your doctor or a therapist.

Although this type of conversation may seem too embarrassing to initiate at first, it can bring positive results in the form of treatment and management of your incontinence. Successful management of your incontinence can increase your confidence in yourself and your ability for sexual expression.

In the meantime, the following suggestions may help improve your sex life:

- *Talk with each other.* As difficult as it may seem initially, talk with your partner about your condition. Obviously, it's important to have a loving partner to begin with, but you may be surprised at how understanding and willing to accommodate your partner can be. In any intimate relationship, regardless of how young or healthy the couple, open communication is probably the most important element in achieving mutual satisfaction. If necessary, seek professional help in breaking down communication barriers between you and your partner.
- *Expand your definition of sex.* There are countless variations on sexual intimacy. Touch can be a good alternative to intercourse. It can simply mean holding each other or sensual massage.
- *Try a different position.* Perhaps a different position makes intercourse easier for you. If you're in a comfortable position, you're more likely to feel free to concentrate on making love and may be less prone to leakage. For women, being on top may provide

better pelvic muscle control. Rear entry may ease pressure on your bladder. Ask your partner about his or her needs and ways that you can also be accommodating.

- *Empty your bladder beforehand.* To reduce your chances of leakage during lovemaking, avoid drinking fluids for an hour or so before sex and empty your bladder immediately before starting.
- *Wear a diaphragm (women).* Because of where a diaphragm sits in the female pelvis, it can provide support to the bladder and urethra and help prevent leakage during sexual intercourse.
- *Do your Kegels.* Pelvic floor muscle exercises (Kegels) can help strengthen your pelvic floor muscles and reduce leakage.
- *Be prepared.* Having towels handy or using disposable pads on your bed may help ease some of your anxiety if you're worried about wetness.
- *Keep a sense of humor.* Remember that sex is rarely as perfect as it appears in the movies. People are human, and if it's not one particular problem, it may be another. A sense of humor can help you overcome problems and even create greater intimacy between you and your partner.

KEEPING A POSITIVE OUTLOOK

Studies have found that depression is frequently associated with incontinence and that incontinence can have a negative effect on quality of life. If your condition is severe, you may begin to withdraw from social situations and isolate yourself from others, including your family, for fear of having an accident or worry that an odor may be present.

Whenever your body doesn't work as it used to or as it should, it's natural to feel a sense of loss, even if the change isn't permanent. Losing control of something that used to be second nature can trigger surprisingly intense feelings of grief, anger and despair.

It's easy to trivialize emotions connected with incontinence because it's not a life-threatening or necessarily painful condition. In fact, many people find it embarrassing to even admit to themselves, let alone to others, that they have the condition.

But when incontinence begins to take a toll on your life, it's important to recognize the emotions that you may feel and to work through them in a healthy way. Your mental outlook is a key factor in learning to manage your condition.

Practicing positive thinking

Positive thinking means that you try to approach the unpleasantness of your situation in a more positive and productive way. Instead of thinking that the worst is going to happen, you try to see things more optimistically.

Positive thinking often starts with what's called self-talk. Self-talk is the endless stream of unspoken thoughts that run through your head every day. These automatic thoughts can be positive or negative. Some of your self-talk comes from logic and reason. Other self-talk may arise from misconceptions that you create because of lack of information.

If the thoughts that run through your head are mostly negative, your outlook on life is likely to be pessimistic. If, on the other hand, your thoughts are mostly positive, you're likely an optimist — someone who practices positive thinking.

To help you develop more of a positive outlook, here are some tips:
- Don't say anything to yourself that you wouldn't say to anyone else. Be gentle and encouraging with yourself. If a negative thought enters your mind, evaluate it rationally and respond with affirmations of what is good about you.
- Periodically during the day, stop and evaluate what you're thinking. If you find that your thoughts are mainly negative, try to find a way to put a positive spin on them.
- Give yourself permission to smile or laugh, especially during difficult times. Seek humor in everyday happenings. When you can laugh at life, you feel less stressed and are better able to cope.
- Surround yourself with positive people. Make sure those in your life are positive, supportive people you can depend on. Negative people may increase your stress level and dampen your mood.

SEEKING HELP

It can't be emphasized enough that help is available for incontinence. Being incontinent is not a normal part of aging, and you don't have to accept it as such, even though your parents or grandparents may have. Treatment is available to cure incontinence or significantly reduce its effect on your life. Even if you have incontinence that's related to another illness or medical condition, in many cases the incontinence can still be effectively treated.

For a successful outcome, the key elements are:
- Finding a doctor who is interested in your condition, will perform a thorough diagnosis and will help you find the best way to treat your type of incontinence. See page 8 for more information on incontinence specialists.
- Being actively involved in your treatment. Treatment for incontinence often involves therapies, whether behavioral or medicinal, that require active participation, commitment and patience on your part.

You might also consider joining a support group. Organizations such as the National Association for Continence (NAFC) can provide you with resources and information about people who experience stress incontinence (see page 188). Support groups offer a venue for voicing concerns and often provide motivation to maintain self-care strategies.

Although achieving bladder control may seem difficult and even impossible at times, don't give up. It's a worthwhile goal, and once you achieve it, you'll find renewed confidence in yourself and your abilities.

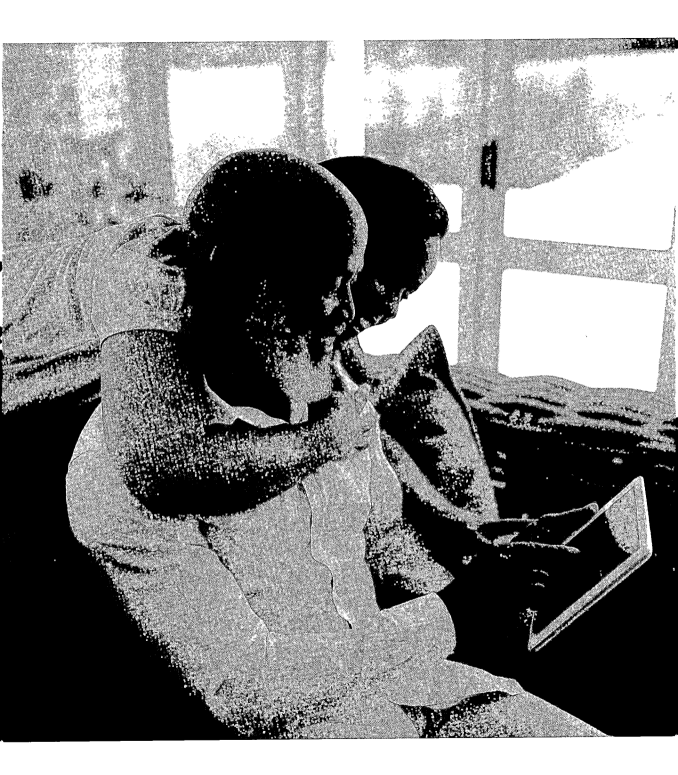

Fecal incontinence

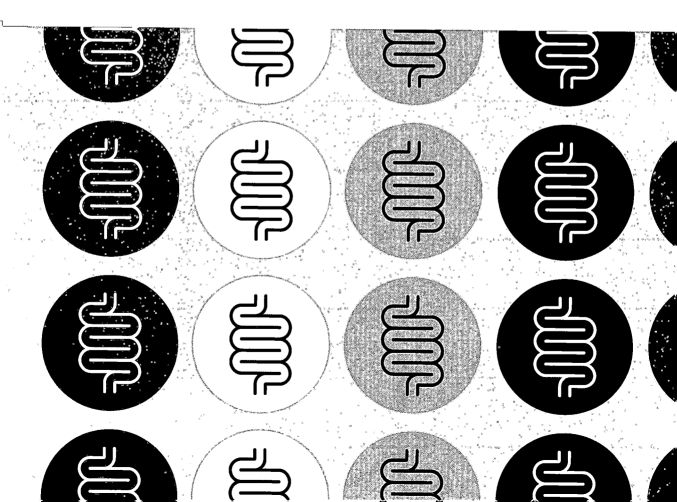

9

Understanding fecal incontinence

Fecal incontinence is not something you hear much about, but it affects a number of people. Fecal incontinence is the inability to control your bowel movements, causing stool (feces) to leak unexpectedly from your rectum. Also called accidental bowel leakage, fecal incontinence ranges from occasional leakage of stool while passing gas to a complete loss of bowel control.

Most of us take bowel control for granted. We generally don't have an "accident" unless we have a short-lived bout of diarrhea. That's not the case for people with recurring (chronic) fecal incontinence. They can't control the passage of gas or stool, which may be liquid or solid.

People with fecal incontinence may also pass gas involuntarily. Although the involuntary passing of gas in itself isn't defined as fecal incontinence, it can be a distressing problem.

Many people with fecal incontinence also have urinary incontinence. This is referred to as double incontinence. Double incontinence is more common among women than men.

Fecal incontinence can have a devastating effect on nearly every aspect of your daily life, including your self-image, your work and your relationships. As you try to manage a bodily process that can't be controlled, your confidence, self-respect and composure can falter. You may feel ashamed, embarrassed or humiliated.

Many people with fecal incontinence are afraid to leave the house in case they have an accident in public. They feel as if they're "tethered to the toilet." It can be hard to take a walk around the block, let alone ride in a car, bus or airplane. Social functions are daunting, to say the least. Keeping a job can be challenging.

Most people with fecal incontinence don't tell anyone about it, not even their doctors. Instead, they limit their activities and withdraw from friends and family. The results can be social isolation, job loss, lowered self-esteem, depression and anxiety.

Fecal incontinence is more common in older people, but it can affect anyone, including children after they've been toilet trained. It's difficult to determine how common the problem is, since many people are reluctant to report it. It's estimated that between 2% and 7% of the general population is affected by fecal incontinence, but the actual incidence may be much higher.

Even though fecal incontinence often affects older people, it's not a normal part of aging. And it's not a hopeless situation, no matter what your age. Improvements in the understanding, awareness, diagnosis and treatment of the problem have brightened the outlook for people with fecal incontinence. Most people can be helped with proper treatment, and often the problem can be completely resolved.

Taking steps to deal with fecal incontinence will help ease the embarrassment, fear, anxiety and loneliness that often come with the physical problems. Treatment can improve your life and help you

feel better about yourself. This chapter will help you understand what causes fecal incontinence, how your bowels work and what happens if something goes wrong.

HOW YOUR BOWELS WORK

Fecal incontinence isn't a specific disease. Rather, it's a sign of one or more medical problems. It can happen when something goes wrong with the complex, coordinated process that allows you to hold stool in until you choose to release it. Fecal incontinence can result for a variety of reasons and is rarely due to a single factor. To understand the causes of fecal incontinence, it's helpful to know something about the way your bowels normally work.

Continence is a function of a healthy digestive system. Your digestive tract begins at your mouth and ends at the rectum and anus in the lower portion of the large intestine. The digestive tract consists of several organs that work together to process the food you eat, absorb vital nutrients and fluids into your bloodstream, and remove waste that your body can't digest.

When your bowels are functioning normally, waste material progresses in an orderly fashion through the last part of the digestive tract — the large intestine (colon), rectum and anus. By the time digested food has reached this point, the nutrients have been absorbed. In the colon, nearly all of the water is removed from the waste. The remaining residue,

The digestive tract begins at the mouth and ends at the rectum. It involves a number of vital internal organs.

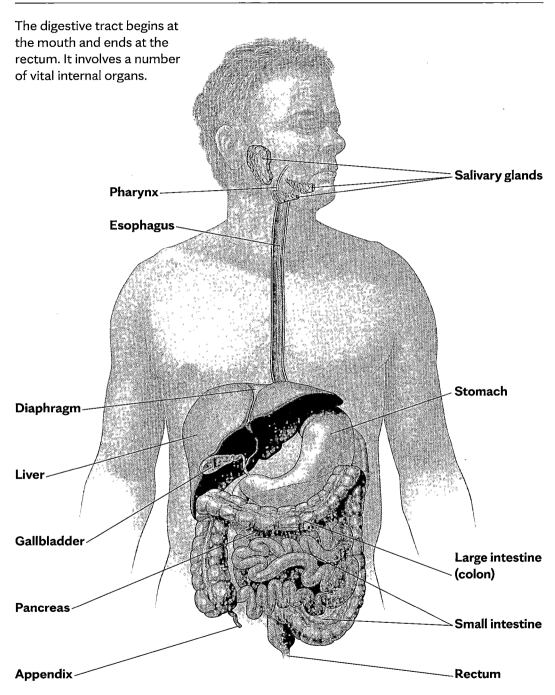

Salivary glands

Pharynx

Esophagus

Stomach

Diaphragm

Liver

Gallbladder

Large intestine (colon)

Pancreas

Small intestine

Appendix

Rectum

called stool (feces), is usually soft but formed. Stool is composed of undigested food, unabsorbed water, bacteria, mucus and dead cells. It's stored in the rectum before being released through the anus.

Bowel function is mainly controlled by three things:
- The strength of your anal sphincters, the ring-like muscles at the end of your rectum. These muscles tighten (contract) to prevent stool from leaving your rectum.
- The storage capacity of your rectum, allowing you to hold stool for some time after you're aware the stool is there.

- The ability to sense the need to pass stool.

To remain continent, your colon, rectum, anus and nervous system all have to be working normally. In addition, you have to be able to recognize and respond to the urge to go to the bathroom. Other factors that play a role include how food and waste move through your colon and the consistency and amount of stool.

The colon

The colon, also called the large intestine or bowel, is about 5 feet long. It extends

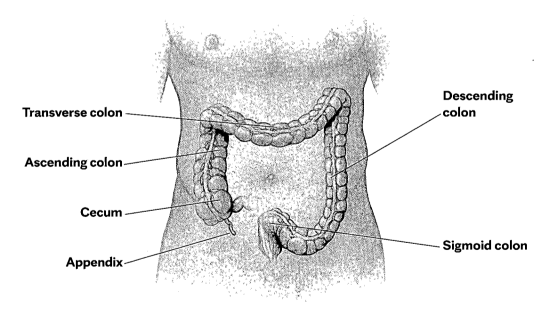

Transverse colon
Ascending colon
Cecum
Appendix
Descending colon
Sigmoid colon

Your colon consists of four sections, beginning at the point where it joins the small intestine at the cecum and ending with the sigmoid section, just above the rectum.

from the point where it joins the small intestine, in the lower right side of your abdomen, up toward the liver. From there it crosses the top of your abdomen, then turns sharply downward along the left side of the abdomen toward your pelvis.

The last sections of the colon — the sigmoid colon, rectum and anus — are crucial to continence.

The lower part of the colon that descends from the top of the pelvic bone to the rectum is called the sigmoid colon. The name refers to its S-shaped curve (from the Greek word *sigma*, or S). The sigmoid colon helps slow the passage of fecal material before it moves into the rectum and then is expelled.

It can take as long as 10 hours to several days for digestive contents to move through the entire colon. As they do, most of the fluid and salts are absorbed from the material. The contents dry out and become more solid and take the form of stool. Stool is stored in the sigmoid colon until muscle contractions move it into the rectum.

These muscle movements, known as peristaltic waves, propel stool forward toward the rectum. Peristaltic waves usually last for about 10 to 15 minutes two or three times a day, most commonly after awakening or after a meal.

Eating increases activity of the colon, causing you to feel like you need to use the bathroom. That's why many people grab the newspaper and head to the bathroom after breakfast.

The rectum and anal canal

The rectum lies at the end of the large intestine, just after the sigmoid colon. The rectum is a hollow muscular tube about 5 inches long. It's more elastic than is the rest of the bowel, so it can expand to store fecal material. Normally, the rectum is empty. When stool is pushed into the rectum from the colon, its walls stretch to accommodate it. The rectum is surrounded by nerves that sense the expansion and trigger the urge to have a bowel movement. As more stool enters the rectum, the urge increases.

As the rectal walls stretch, the internal anal sphincter muscle relaxes. The internal anal sphincter is one of two circular layers of muscle surrounding the last 2 inches of the rectum, called the anal canal (see the illustration on page 130). The anal canal ends at the anus — the opening at the end of the digestive tract.

Most of the time, the internal anal sphincter stays tightened (contracted) to prevent leakage from the rectum into the anal canal. But when the rectum expands, the internal anal sphincter opens briefly and lets a tiny bit of the rectum's contents come into contact with the many nerve endings in the anal canal. In a rapid "sampling reflex," sensory nerve receptors detect whether the rectal contents are gas or liquid or solid stool. This allows you to decide what to do — pass gas or hold in the stool.

If you have diarrhea or loose stool, you'll want to get to a bathroom quickly. If your stool is solid, you may wait for a more convenient time or place to use the bathroom.

Stool is held in the rectum by the external anal sphincter muscle. As your rectum expands, the external sphincter muscle tightens.

This is a unique muscle in that it can be tightened two ways. You can consciously constrict the muscle to hold stool in while you get to a bathroom. The external sphincter can also hold in stool by reflex, without conscious control. For example, when you're sleeping, the internal and external anal sphincters stay contracted to keep stool from leaving the rectum. This reflex also kicks in when you cough, laugh heartily or lift something heavy so that the sudden increase in pressure in your abdomen doesn't force stool out.

Holding stool

If you need to delay having a bowel movement, you tighten your external anal sphincter. You also contract the puborectalis muscle in your pelvic floor. This U-shaped muscle forms a sling that supports the area between the rectum and the anal canal. When the muscle is contracted, it pulls the rectum so that it lies at an angle — above and to the side of the anal canal, rather than straight above it. This prevents stool from passing from the rectum into the anal canal.

You can actively tighten your external sphincter muscle for only a few minutes at the most. After that, your rectum stretches to hold more stool, the sense of urgency gradually subsides and the external sphincter relaxes. The internal anal sphincter closes, keeping stool in the rectum.

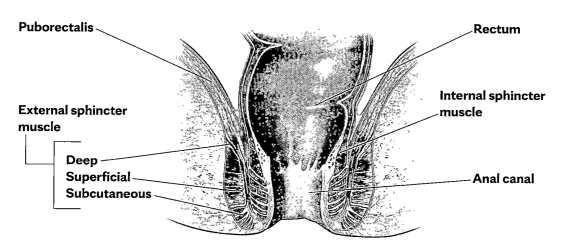

Puborectalis　　　　　　　　　　　　　　　**Rectum**

External sphincter muscle

Deep
Superficial
Subcutaneous

Internal sphincter muscle

Anal canal

The external and internal anal sphincter muscles work together with the muscles of the rectum to control the passage of stool. When the anal sphincter muscles are damaged or weakened, fecal incontinence may result.

The rectum's ability to stretch and store stool is known as compliance. Of course, there comes a point when the rectum is holding all the stool it can and you feel an urgent need to go to the bathroom. Generally, the rectum can hold up to about 10 ounces (a little over 1 cup) of stool before things get uncomfortable.

Moving your bowels

When you're ready to have a bowel movement, all the muscles involved in maintaining continence — the internal and external anal sphincters and the puborectalis — relax.

When you sit or squat, the angle between the anus and rectum straightens, allowing feces in the rectum to move into the anus. As you push, your external anal sphincter and puborectalis muscles relax, further straightening the angle (see below).

To propel stool downward, you may bear down — what's called the Valsalva maneuver. This closes off the airway, tightens the abdominal muscles and pushes the diaphragm down. The Valsalva maneuver increases pressure in the abdomen, helping to empty the rectum.

FECAL INCONTINENCE

For your bowels to function normally and keep you from experiencing unintended bowel movements, all of the different, interconnected structures described earlier in this chapter have to be working together. Think of the digestive tract as something like a factory production line — various organs perform various

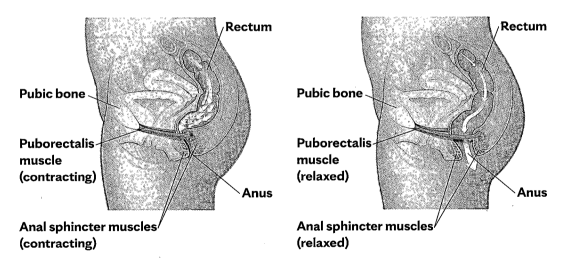

When the puborectalis muscle contracts (left), it holds the rectum at an angle so that stool is prevented from passing into the anal canal. As the muscle relaxes (right), the angle changes, allowing stool to move into the anal canal.

Fecal incontinence can affect men and women, young and old. Even people who don't have fecal incontinence may have an occasional "accident" when they have the stomach flu or other infectious disease that causes diarrhea.

Some factors increase your likelihood of incontinence, however. They include the following:
- Being unable to perform daily living activities, such as dressing yourself or going to the bathroom on your own
- Growing older
- Having chronic diarrhea or constipation
- Being in poor general health
- Giving birth, especially if you've had large babies, a long second stage of delivery, forceps deliveries, breech birth, a cut to extend the vaginal opening (episiotomy) or a vaginal tear that reached the anus
- Having colon, rectal, anal or gynecologic problems
- Taking certain medications, such as laxatives or antacids
- Experiencing late or interrupted toilet training in childhood

In addition, certain diseases and conditions increase your risk of fecal incontinence. They include:
- Diabetes
- Stroke
- Multiple sclerosis
- Parkinson's disease
- Systemic sclerosis
- Myotonic dystrophy
- Amyloidosis
- Spinal cord injuries
- Imperforate anus
- Hirschsprung's disease
- Pelvic organ prolapse and rectal prolapse

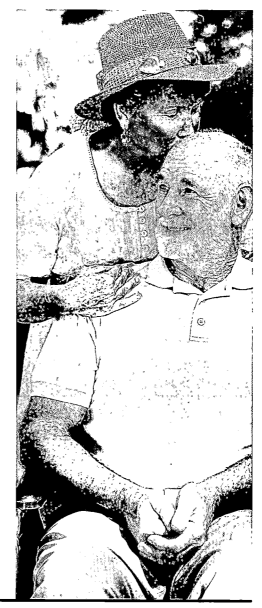

functions at certain sites to process food and fluids into stool. If any part of the line breaks down or stops working — in other words, if part of the system is affected by disease or injury — incontinence may result. Often, more than one factor is involved.

Sometimes, incontinence occurs when an unrelated condition, such as arthritis, makes it physically difficult to reach the toilet in time. This is referred to as functional incontinence.

Causes of fecal incontinence

Common causes of fecal incontinence include recurring (chronic) constipation, diarrhea, and muscle or nerve damage. Muscle damage is involved in most cases of fecal incontinence.

The muscles and nerves in and around the rectum and anus interact to sense the presence of waste, allow it to be stored, propel it along and, finally, eliminate it. Damage to the anal sphincter muscles can result in incontinence. If the muscles are weakened and they can't close tightly, stool leaks out.

The pelvic floor muscles also play an important role in maintaining continence. These muscles support the organs within the pelvis and lower abdomen. If the pelvic floor muscles become weak or their function is disturbed, fecal incontinence can result.

Nerve damage also may be a factor. To remain continent, a person must be able to recognize and respond to the urge to defecate. Conditions that affect your nervous system or cause nerve damage may decrease your awareness or sensation of bowel fullness. If the nerves that control the sphincter muscles are injured, they won't work properly and incontinence can occur. If the nerves that sense stool in the rectum are damaged, you may not feel the need to use the bathroom until stool has leaked out.

A broad range of conditions and disorders can cause fecal incontinence.

Constipation

It's ironic, but the most common cause of fecal incontinence is constipation. That's because chronic constipation may lead to impacted stool — a large mass of dry, hard stool within your rectum. This mass can be too large for you to pass, and as a result, the muscles of your rectum and intestines stretch, and then eventually weaken. Watery stool from farther up in the digestive system may move around the mass and leak out, causing incontinence.

Constipation is defined as passing stools less frequently than every three days, or excessive straining when trying to move the bowels. While many people believe that they should have at least one bowel movement a day, frequency varies from one person to another. If you pass at least three stools a week without straining, you're probably not constipated.

When constipation occurs frequently (chronic constipation) the anal sphincter muscles become stretched and they weaken. This can cause the nerves of the anus and rectum to become less responsive to the presence of stool.

Chronic constipation may also weaken colon muscles. The result is that transit time in the bowel slows down, making it difficult to pass stools and worsening constipation.

Possible causes of constipation include:
• Lack of physical activity
• Lack of dietary fiber
• Pregnancy and childbirth
• Diabetes and other hormone-related diseases
• Certain medications
• Surgery
• Irritable bowel syndrome
• Repeatedly ignoring the urge to pass stool
• Diseases that affect the nerves, such as multiple sclerosis, stroke, dementia and Parkinson's disease
• Rectal prolapse and rectocele

Diarrhea

Loose stool (diarrhea) is more difficult to control than formed, solid stool. Diarrhea can overwhelm your body's ability to hold stool in. It may be due to many things, including infectious illnesses such as food poisoning or stomach flu. Diarrhea can result from certain medications, including the overuse of laxatives.

Chronic conditions such as inflammatory bowel disease (Crohn's disease and ulcerative colitis) and irritable bowel syndrome can result in diarrhea. Other diseases that affect the colon or rectum, such as diverticular disease and cancer, can cause diarrhea. Radiation therapy is another possible cause.

Muscle damage

Often, the cause of fecal incontinence is injury to the anal sphincter — the rings of muscle at the end of the rectum that help hold in stool. If these muscles are damaged, they're simply not strong enough to hold stool back properly, and some stool may leak out.

This kind of damage can occur during childbirth. The risk of muscle damage is greatest if you tear an anal muscle during delivery.

Other factors that increase the likelihood of muscle damage include the use of forceps during delivery, having a large baby, going through a long second stage of delivery, having to make a cut to enlarge the vaginal opening for delivery (episiotomy) and having a breech birth.

Nerve damage

Fecal incontinence may be associated with damage to the sensory nerves that detect stool in the rectum or to those nerves that control the anal sphincter. Nerve damage can result from childbirth, constant straining during bowel movements, a spinal cord injury or a stroke.

Fecal incontinence isn't an inevitable part of aging. For most people, bowel function remains vigorous and healthy well into old age. But some of the bodily changes that occur with aging can contribute to incontinence.

Over time, your anal sphincter muscles and the muscles and ligaments that support your pelvis can weaken. Older women are especially prone to loss of strength in these areas, most likely because female reproductive hormones influence the strength and vigor of the pelvic floor and anal muscles. After menopause, when a woman's hormone levels drop sharply, the external anal sphincter loses some of its ability to squeeze. In women, the effects of child-birth on the pelvic floor and anal muscles may become apparent only in their later years.

Aging can also bring other changes that may affect bowel function. Changes in the intestinal walls and blood supply slow down the time it takes for food and waste to move through your intestines. You might notice your stools becoming harder and drier and experience more problems with constipation.

Diet and lifestyle also have a significant impact on how well your bowels work as you age. Older adults tend to drink fewer fluids because their sense of thirst is less acute. You also may not eat as well and you may be less physically active than you once were. Constipation can occur if there's not enough fluid or fiber in your diet. Reduced physical activity also increases your risk of constipation.

Diseases that are common in older people, such as diabetes and Parkinson's disease, can contribute to fecal incontinence. Older adults also tend to take more medications, which may result in fecal incontinence.

Diseases such as diabetes and multiple sclerosis can affect rectal and anal nerves and impair their ability to sense or hold stool in the rectum.

Habitual straining when passing stool also can damage the nerves that sense stool in your rectum, in addition to the muscles that support your pelvic organs.

Loss of storage capacity

Normally, your rectum stretches to accommodate stool. If your rectum is scarred or your rectal walls have stiffened from surgery, radiation treatment or inflammatory bowel disease, the rectum can't stretch as much as needed and stool may leak out.

Fecal incontinence is often associated with irritable bowel syndrome (IBS). IBS is characterized by abdominal pain or cramping and changes in bowel pattern, such as loose or more frequent bowel movements, diarrhea, and constipation. It's not completely clear what causes IBS, but symptoms appear to result from a disturbance in the interaction between the intestines, the brain and the part of the nervous system that enables involuntary responses (autonomic nervous system). The result is a colon that's more sensitive and reactive to things such as stress and certain foods.

For most people with IBS, the signs and symptoms are mild. However, IBS can cause frequent diarrhea and constipation, both of which can lead to fecal incontinence. IBS can also lead to reduced storage capacity and sensation in the rectum.

For some people with IBS, the muscle contractions that move food through the digestive tract may be stronger and last longer than normal. Food is forced through your intestines more quickly, causing gas, bloating and diarrhea. This type of IBS is called diarrhea-predominant IBS. Some people with IBS have the opposite problem — food passage slows, and stools become hard and dry, causing constipation. This is known as constipation-predominant IBS.

A few people have alternating bouts of constipation and diarrhea, called mixed IBS. IBS can also produce a sense of straining, urgency or a feeling that you can't empty your bowels completely.

Medications

Some medications can increase your risk of constipation or diarrhea, both of which can lead to incontinence. See page 186 for list of problematic medications.

Surgery

Surgery to treat enlarged veins in the rectum or anus (hemorrhoids) can dam-age the anus and cause fecal incontinence, as can complex operations involving the rectum and anus, or the prostate gland or gynecologic organs.

Scarring of rectum

It can be difficult to hold stool if the rectal walls lose elasticity, becoming stiffer and less able to stretch. This can occur as a result of scarring from rectal surgery, radiation treatment or inflammatory bowel disease.

Rectal cancer

Cancer of the anus and rectum can lead to fecal incontinence if the cancer invades the muscle walls or disrupts the nerve impulses needed for defecation.

Other conditions

If your rectum drops down into your anus (rectal prolapse) or, in women, if the rectum pushes on and causes a bulging of the vagina (rectocele), fecal incontinence can result. People born with conditions affecting the anus or rectum may have lifelong issues with fecal incontinence.

TYPES

When you sense a bowel movement and you aren't able to hold the stool in your rectum long enough to reach a bathroom, it's called urge (active) fecal incontinence. When you experience stool leakage that occurred without any urge to move your bowels, it's known as unsensed (passive) fecal incontinence. Overflow incontinence is a type of fecal incontinence that's associated with constipation.

Urge fecal incontinence

When your external anal sphincter muscle isn't functioning properly, you may not be able to hold stool in your rectum. As soon as you sense stool in your rectum, you feel an urgent need to go to the bathroom. And you may not be able to squeeze the sphincter muscle hard enough or long enough to reach the toilet in time.

Childbirth is a common cause of anal sphincter damage. Vaginal birth can cause tears in both the internal and external anal sphincter muscles, as well as damage to the pudendal nerve, the major nerve to the external sphincter. Some women develop fecal incontinence within weeks of giving birth. For others, the problem doesn't show up until they're in their mid-40s or older, when the muscles and supporting structures in the pelvis can weaken.

Other causes of anal sphincter damage include surgery to the rectal or anal area, including surgery for hemorrhoids. Injury to the anal area and loss of anal muscle strength are additional culprits. Aging is also a significant factor.

Individuals with damage to the nerves in the pelvic floor may have problems with the rectum being able to accommodate stool. Stool passes through the sigmoid colon and rectum very quickly, and the barriers that normally hold stool in may become overwhelmed. This can result in diarrhea or a lack of time between first sensing the presence of stool in the rectum and having an urgent need to use the bathroom. This type of nerve damage may occur from diabetes, multiple sclerosis, or spinal cord or brain injuries.

A sense of urgency and frequent bowel movements can also occur if your rectum can't stretch enough to store a normal amount of stool. Normally the rectum stretches to hold stool until you can get to a bathroom. But if your rectum can't stretch as it should, you'll have less time between sensing the presence of stool and the urgent need to use the bathroom.

Even if your anal sphincter muscles are working properly, you may experience fecal incontinence if your rectum has become stiff. Your rectum may also not be able to hold as much stool as normal as a result of scarring from surgery, pelvic radiation or inflammatory bowel disease.

A condition called rectal prolapse can make you feel an urgent need to go even when little stool is present. Rectal prolapse happens when the muscles supporting the rectum are weak, and the rectum shifts downward into the anal canal or out of the body (prolapses). If you have rectal prolapse, your external sphincter must work harder to hold stool in. Prolapse can cause sphincter muscle damage.

Unsensed fecal incontinence

Rectal sensation tells you that stool is in your rectum and that you need to get to a bathroom. If the nerves that are responsible for sensation in your rectum or anus are damaged, you may lose the ability to sense stool in your rectum. Or you may not be able to distinguish between gas, solid stool and liquid stool.

If your rectal sensation is impaired, you may not recognize the need to have a bowel movement. You may pass stool involuntarily, or excessive stool may accumulate in your rectum. This can cause impacted stool, hard fecal matter that's stuck in the rectum.

Causes of impaired rectal sensation include nerve damage from diabetes, multiple sclerosis, stroke and spinal cord injury. Nerve injury can also occur from childbirth or from years of hard straining to have a bowel movement. Some medications, such as opiate (narcotic) painkillers and antidepressants, also can affect rectal sensation and lead to fecal incontinence. Rectal sensation may be blunted in older adults and in physically and mentally challenged individuals.

Damage to your internal anal sphincter muscle can lead to bits of stool leaking out without you being aware of it. A poor "seal" in the muscle allows stool to leak. If the sphincter sampling reflex is impaired, you may not be able to determine the contents of the rectum and decide what to do. The same things that can damage the external anal sphincter — childbirth, injury, surgery, muscle weakness with age — can also cause problems with the internal sphincter.

The ability to sense stool in the rectum also requires that a person is alert enough to notice the sensation and do something about it. A person with dementia may not notice the sensation. Fecal incontinence is often an aspect of late-stage Alzheimer's disease, in which both dementia and nerve damage play a role.

Overflow incontinence

Overflow incontinence refers to the type of incontinence that commonly accompanies constipation.

With overflow incontinence a large mass of dry, hard stool may form in the rectum and the mass becomes too large to pass. The stuck (impacted) stool causes your internal anal sphincter muscle to stretch and weaken. Meanwhile, watery stool from higher in the bowel may move around the mass of stool and leak out. The watery stool may look like diarrhea, but it doesn't occur for the same reasons as diarrhea.

A HOPEFUL OUTLOOK

Many people aren't aware that fecal incontinence can be treated. You don't have to suffer in silence. Several different therapies are available that address the various causes. Treatment can improve your bowel control, and coping strategies can make living with fecal incontinence a little easier.

Working up the courage to admit that you have the problem is the first step in managing it. The following chapters provide information about getting help for fecal incontinence and about the different types of treatments.

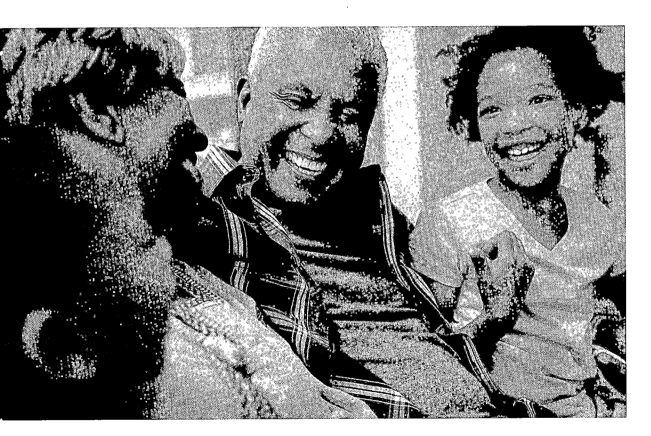

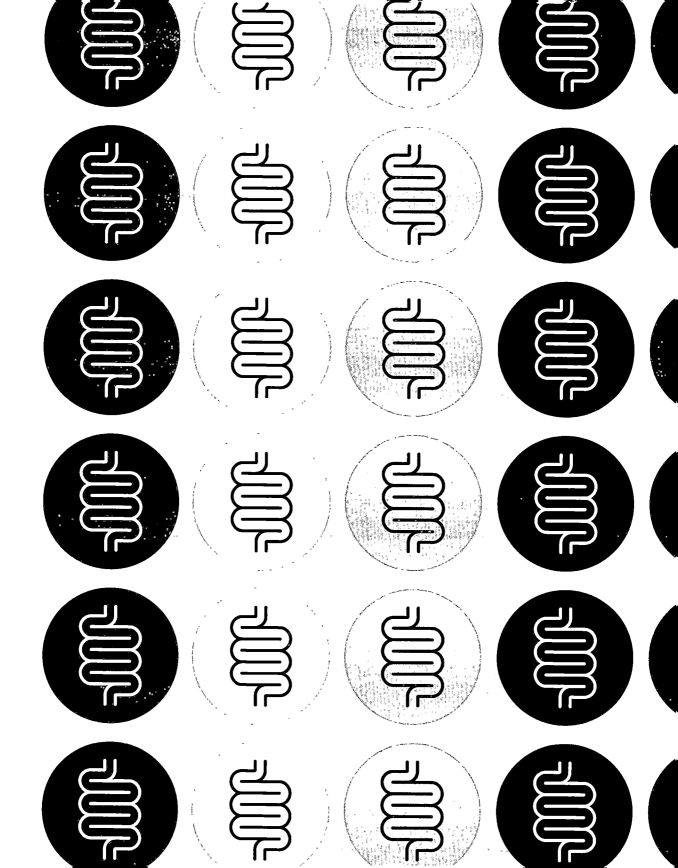

CHAPTER

Evaluation and testing

10

Many people who live with fecal incontinence typically carry an added burden of shame and secrecy. They're embarrassed to tell a doctor about the problem. They may not realize that fecal incontinence is treatable, or they've had a bad experience with a doctor who didn't provide useful solutions or compassionate care.

Some people try to cope on their own — buying adult diapers, memorizing every toilet facility in a given area, bringing a change of clothes every time they go out. These strategies work to a degree, but if you rely only on them, you may miss out on more effective treatments. Not getting help can result in needless anxiety and stress.

Don't shy away from talking to your doctor about fecal incontinence. Many

treatments — some of which are very simple — that can improve, if not cure, incontinence are available. Nearly everyone can be helped in some way.

To your doctor, fecal incontinence isn't a personal problem or a reflection of your abilities, control or worth. It's a medical condition that needs to be investigated and treated. Ideally, your doctor will be your ally as you work together to find the best approach to your condition.

CHOOSING A DOCTOR

To get help for fecal incontinence, you might start with your primary care provider. Not all primary care providers are familiar with evaluating and treating fecal incontinence, though. You may need to see someone who specializes in treating conditions that affect the colon, rectum and anus.

Several types of medical professionals work with people who have fecal incontinence, including:

- *Gastroenterologists.* A gastroenterologist is trained to treat conditions of the digestive (gastrointestinal) tract, including fecal incontinence. If you have diarrhea or digestive symptoms in addition to incontinence, consider seeing a gastroenterologist.
- *Colorectal surgeons.* A colorectal surgeon provides surgical and nonsurgical treatment for conditions that affect the colon, rectum and anus.
- *Female pelvic medicine and reconstructive surgery specialists.* A specialist with these credentials is an obstetrician-gynecologist (OB-GYN) or a urologist who's had additional training in diseases and disorders affecting the bladder and pelvis in women, including urinary and fecal incontinence.

Some medical facilities that specialize in evaluating people with fecal incontinence will have what's known as an anorectal physiology lab. The lab has trained clinicians and the necessary equipment for performing tests used to investigate possible causes of fecal incontinence.

What to expect

When you meet with a doctor to talk about fecal incontinence, it's important to feel comfortable. You have the right to be treated with dignity and respect. If the doctor seems to dismiss your problem, suggests that you use pads or tells you there's not much that can be done, find another physician.

Ask your doctor about his or her experience in treating fecal incontinence and about the range of treatments available. Not all doctors are aware that the problem is often correctable. Look for an individual who listens to your concerns, answers your questions and explains things clearly. He or she should show concern about how incontinence is affecting your quality of life.

EVALUATING FECAL INCONTINENCE

The answers you provide to questions during your initial appointment will help establish the degree and frequency of your problem and its impact on your life. You will likely be asked many health-related questions, followed by a physical examination. Additional tests may be needed to confirm the diagnosis. An accurate understanding of the cause or causes of your condition is essential for planning treatment.

Medical history

Your doctor will likely ask many questions about your symptoms, medical history and lifestyle. A thorough medical history can provide many clues about the origins of incontinence. Some medical institutions use a standardized questionnaire or form to gather the information and grade the severity of the incontinence.

QUESTIONS YOU MAY BE ASKED DURING YOUR EXAM

During your initial evaluation, your doctor will likely ask a lot of detailed questions about your bowel habits. Although you may find it embarrassing to reveal such personal information, it can help point toward what's causing the problem and what tests may be needed.

Be prepared to answer the following questions:

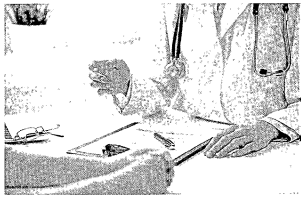

- When did the incontinence start?
- How often do you lose control of your bowels? What happens — do you lose a small or large amount of stool? Is it liquid or solid? Do you have any warning?
- Do you know when your rectum is full? Are you able to distinguish between gas and stool? Do you sometimes think you're passing gas and then are surprised to find that stool has come out?
- Does anything seem to bring on the incontinence, such as physical activity, illness, stress or specific foods? Does anything seem to make it better or worse?
- Has the problem gotten worse over time? Did it start after a particular event, such as surgery or childbirth?
- Do you experience incontinence at certain times of the day? Does it happen only at night or during the day? After meals? After a bowel movement?
- When you feel the need to have a bowel movement, how long can you wait?
- After you defecate, do you feel like there's stool left inside?
- What are your regular bowel habits? Have there been changes in your bowel habits over the years?
- Do you often have diarrhea or constipation? Do you have to strain to pass stool? Is there any discomfort? Do you have cramps or see blood in your stool?
- Do you also experience urinary incontinence?
- Do you use pads or other devices to cope with incontinence? How is that working?
- Do you use anything to help with bowel movements, such as laxatives, enemas or suppositories?
- What medications are you taking?
- What is your typical diet?
- How does incontinence affect your life and how you feel about yourself?

The purpose of the questionnaire is to help determine whether you have true fecal incontinence and how severe it is. Expect questions about when the incontinence started, how often it occurs, whether the stool is liquid or solid, and whether you're aware of the need to go to the bathroom before the incontinence occurs. You may be asked to describe your normal bowel habits.

Women are often asked about their history of childbirth, including the length of their labors, how much their babies weighed, whether they had a breech birth, whether the deliveries required forceps or episiotomies, whether they had any tears that needed repair, and how their bowels functioned afterward.

Your doctor may ask you if you also have urinary incontinence, since urinary and fecal incontinence are sometimes related. He or she may want to know if you've had surgery, injuries or radiation treatment in your pelvic region or any back or spinal cord injuries. You may be asked about any other medical conditions you have, such as diabetes or irritable bowel syndrome.

Let your doctor know about any medications you take. Certain medications may cause or increase the frequency of fecal incontinence (see page 186). Your doctor may also ask you about your diet and how much caffeine you consume.

It's important to talk about how you're coping with the incontinence and how it affects your daily life, relationships and self-esteem. Let your doctor know if you've made adjustments in your behav-

ior or lifestyle, such as using pads, carrying a change of clothes or not going out much to avoid the embarrassment of losing bowel control.

Your doctor may ask you to keep a diary of your symptoms and bowel habits. (See page 184 for an example of a bowel diary that you can copy and use.) Some items that might be recorded include bowel movements; incontinence episodes; the consistency of the stool; any feelings of straining, discomfort or incomplete emptying; and use of enemas or laxatives.

Physical exam

Your initial visit will also likely include a physical examination. A physical exam can identify an injury or structural problem in the anal and rectal area, such as rectal prolapse, rectocele or fecal impaction. An exam may also help determine if the fecal incontinence stems from another problem, such as an ulcer or nerve damage from diseases such as diabetes or Parkinson's.

To check for signs of neurological disease or damage, your doctor may examine your reflexes, walking gait and senses. He or she may also feel your abdomen. Swelling, tenderness or pain in your abdomen may indicate gas, fluid or a blockage of some kind in your colon.

A rectal examination is necessary to evaluate fecal incontinence. Some people consider this exam uncomfortable and undignified, but it provides a great amount of information that can be key to diagnosing your condition. A rectal exam also helps your provider determine if additional tests are needed.

A rectal exam generally starts with a visual inspection of your anus and the area between your anus and genitals, called the perineum. Your doctor looks for fecal matter, hemorrhoids, reddening, scarring and signs of infection. Your buttocks are gently spread apart, and the shape of your anus is checked — open or closed, round or asymmetrical, intact or showing signs of skin tearing.

Sensation in the area between your anus and genitals may be checked. Using a pin, probe or cotton swab, your doctor gently touches various points around your anus to see if it puckers up — a "winking" reflex that occurs as the anal sphincter contracts. This test helps check for nerve damage.

Your provider then inserts a gloved, lubricated finger into your rectum to evaluate the strength of your sphincter muscles and to feel for hemorrhoids, growths, tears or protrusions (see below). This part of the exam can also identify a large mass of hard stool within your rectum (fecal impaction). Impaction can lead to overflow incontinence, in which watery stool leaks out around the mass.

During a rectal exam you may be asked to squeeze your anal muscles around your doctor's finger, as if you were trying to hold back gas or delay having a bowel movement. This can help determine whether the rectal sphincter muscles and the puborectalis muscle in your pelvic floor are working — is there a resting muscle tone, can you generate an extra squeeze, can you relax your muscles, do the muscles keep the colon and rectum at the proper angle?

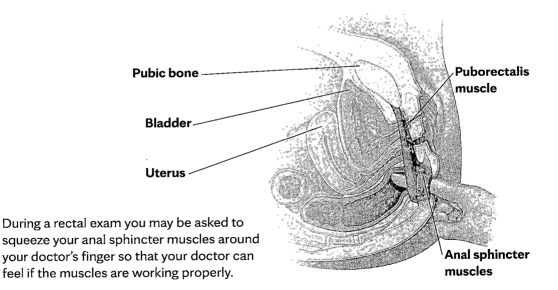

Pubic bone

Bladder

Uterus

Puborectalis muscle

Anal sphincter muscles

During a rectal exam you may be asked to squeeze your anal sphincter muscles around your doctor's finger so that your doctor can feel if the muscles are working properly.

This exam can also help identify rectal prolapse, a condition in which the rectum drops down into the anus. If your doctor suspects rectal prolapse, he or she may ask you to sit upright on a toilet and strain and lean forward while he or she inspects your anal area.

If you feel pain during the rectal exam, tell your doctor. The exam may be uncomfortable, but it shouldn't be painful.

TESTS FOR FECAL INCONTINENCE

The findings of your medical history and the results of the physical exam may uncover the cause of your problem and determine the course of treatment, which may include dietary changes or changes in your fluid intake or the medications you take. Your doctor may also recom-

mend pelvic floor muscle exercises. See Chapter 11 for more information.

More often, though, additional information is needed to pinpoint the cause of fecal incontinence and make an accurate diagnosis.

A number of tests are used to investigate the possible causes of incontinence. Imaging tests provide a visual picture of the lower colon, rectum and anus. Functional tests assess how well certain systems are working. The type of tests you may receive will depend on your symptoms, medical history and physical exam.

Manometry

Manometry, also called anal manometry or anorectal manometry, is the most com-

IF YOU HAVE DIARRHEA OR CONSTIPATION

If you have diarrhea along with fecal incontinence, your doctor may ask you for a stool sample. It will be tested in the laboratory for bacteria or other organisms that could cause infection. Your doctor may also want to examine your rectum and colon using a flexible viewing tube (scope) to make sure the diarrhea isn't associated with inflammation in the colon or a mass in the rectum (see page 149.)

If you're experiencing ongoing constipation, your doctor may perform colon transit studies. These tests check whether digestive contents are moving through your colon too slowly. To prepare for the test, stop taking all laxatives three days beforehand. The procedure involves swallowing a slightly radioactive tracer substance that follows the journey from mouth to anus. The markers within the substance can be seen on X-rays, indicting how long it takes them to travel through the digestive tract.

monly used test for evaluating fecal incontinence.

This test measures the pressure inside your rectum and anal sphincters. It checks the strength of your anal sphincter muscles and their ability to relax and tighten at the proper times. It also evaluates the sensitivity and function of your rectum.

The test may be done in your doctor's office or at a clinic or hospital. It takes about 30 minutes to an hour. As you're lying on your side, a narrow, flexible tube about the circumference of a rectal thermometer is inserted into your anus and rectum. The tube has a small, deflated balloon at the end. Once the tube is in place, the balloon may be expanded.

The balloon senses the pressure inside your rectum, your internal anal sphincter and your external anal sphincter and then transmits the data to a computer. The results are displayed on a graph that looks something like that of a polygraph.

Pressure measurements are recorded as you rest, squeeze and bear down as if trying to pass stool. An abnormally low sphincter pressure indicates a problem with a muscle. Decreased pressure when you're resting or relaxed suggests a problem with the internal anal sphincter, and decreased pressure when you're squeezing suggests that the external anal sphincter isn't working properly.

Manometry is also used to check sensation in your rectum. The ability to sense stool in your rectum is critical for being able to know when you need to go to the bathroom. The test also evaluates how well your rectum expands and contracts when stool enters it.

You may be asked to close your eyes as the balloon is inflated. As the balloon fills with air or fluid, a member of the medical team will ask you to indicate when you can sense the balloon filling. During the examination you may also be asked to indicate when you feel the first sensation in your rectum, when you feel an urge to defecate and when the sensation starts to feel urgent.

A computer records the changes in pressure in your rectum as the balloon is expanded to different levels. This reflects the rectum's ability to stretch.

Balloon expulsion

The balloon expulsion test is another test often performed during manometry. Most people with fecal incontinence are able to have normal bowel movements, but individuals whose fecal incontinence is caused by chronic constipation and impacted stool may have trouble passing stool normally.

A balloon expulsion test evaluates bowel function and your basic ability to defecate. More precisely, it evaluates the ability of your puborectalis muscle to relax and the coordination of your abdominal, pelvic floor and anal sphincter muscles. The test involves expelling the balloon that's been placed in your rectum.

Your doctor may want to use a viewing instrument to take a closer look at your anus, rectum and colon. This enables him or her to see signs of disease or other problems that could cause fecal incontinence, such as inflammation, a tumor, scar tissue or rectal prolapse.

He or she is looking for changes in the lining of your colon and rectum that might reflect damage to underlying nerves and muscles. Visual examination is also useful for evaluating diarrhea, constipation or other changes in bowel habits.

Two procedures are used to view the colon and rectum — proctosigmoidoscopy and colonoscopy. Together the tests are referred to as lower gastrointestinal endoscopy. Colonoscopy isn't usually necessary for evaluating fecal incontinence, but your doctor may suggest it if your symptoms point to the possibility of colorectal cancer or another disease of the colon.

Both tests use a long, slender tube with a tiny video camera and light on the end. The tube is attached to a video monitor. The camera provides a clear, detailed view of the lining of the colon and rectum. The doctor can see bleeding, inflammation, abnormal growths or ulcers.

For proctosigmoidoscopy, a tube called a sigmoidoscope is used to examine your rectum and sigmoid colon, and perhaps part of your descending colon. Colonoscopy is performed using a colonoscope, a tube that's long enough to inspect the full length of the large intestine and part of the small intestine.

Your colon and rectum must be completely empty during these procedures. The night before, you'll be asked to drink only clear liquids, and you won't be able to eat or drink anything after midnight. You'll cleanse your bowels by taking a laxative or having an enema.

The test is done on an outpatient basis at a hospital or in your doctor's office. A proctosigmoidoscopy takes 10 to 20 minutes. A colonoscopy takes 30 to 60 minutes. For a colonoscopy, you'll be given medication to make you relaxed and drowsy.

For both exams, you'll lie on your left side on an examining table. The doctor will gently insert the well-lubricated scope into your rectum and slowly guide it into your colon. You may feel as if you need to move your bowels as the scope is advanced. The scope can be used to blow air into the colon and rectum to inflate them, which allows for a better view of the lining. You may feel some cramping or fullness as this happens.

If your doctor discovers anything unusual, such as a small growth on the lining of the colon (polyp) or inflamed tissue, he or she may remove a piece of it using instruments inserted into the scope. The tissue sample (biopsy) can be tested for cell abnormalities. After the test, you can get back to your usual diet and activities right away. You may pass gas or feel some mild bloating or cramping. These symptoms usually disappear within a day.

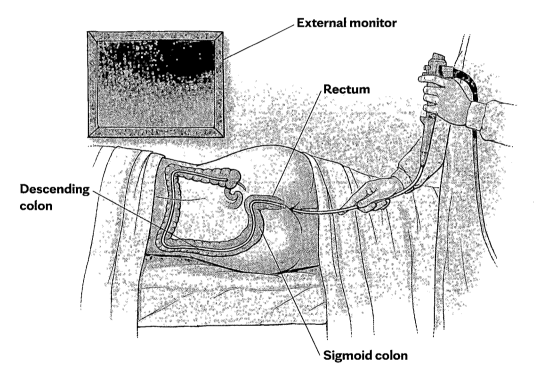

External monitor

Rectum

Descending colon

Sigmoid colon

During colonoscopy a flexible endoscope is inserted into your rectum and threaded through the length of your colon. Images of the lower gastrointestinal tract appear on an external monitor.

Ultrasound

Ultrasound uses sound waves to create images of the internal and external anal sphincters. Anal ultrasound is used to evaluate the structure of the anal sphincters and can identify defects, scarring, thinning or other abnormalities in these muscles.

This imaging test may be referred to by various names — endoanal ultrasonography, endorectal ultrasonography, anorectal ultrasonography and endosonography.

For the test, a probe that emits sound waves is placed on the tip of a flexible or rigid viewing tube called an endoscope. The ultrasound probe, which is attached to a computer and video screen, is inserted through your anus and into your rectum. The waves bounce off the walls of your rectum and anus, producing video images of these internal structures. The doctor can see how your sphincter muscles move and whether any part of them is torn, missing or too thin.

Anal ultrasound is most useful for identifying sphincter injuries or defects and ruling out other muscle or nerve damage as the cause of incontinence. If your medical history suggests that you may have a tear or other problem in the anal sphincters, your doctor will likely recommend this test.

Anal electromyography

If the nerves that control your anal sphincter muscles are damaged, the muscles may not work properly, leading to fecal incontinence. Fecal incontinence is often the result of both muscle and nerve damage. For example, childbirth can injure the pudendal nerve — the major nerve supplying the external anal sphincter — as well as the sphincter muscles.

Anal electromyography (EMG) can assess whether nerve damage is causing or contributing to fecal incontinence. The test may be useful if you have an underlying disease, such as diabetes, that may cause nerve damage or if your doctor believes that you may have pelvic floor nerve damage from childbirth, surgery or an injury. Assessing the extent of nerve damage can help determine whether surgery is likely to be helpful.

Anal EMG records electrical activity within your anal sphincter muscles. For this test, a small sponge containing an electrode is inserted into your anus. It's similar to having a digital rectal exam, with the addition of the sponge electrode attached to your doctor's gloved finger. As you squeeze and relax your sphincter muscles, the electrode will record their electrical signals.

Less commonly, the test may be done with tiny needle electrodes inserted into muscles around your anus. However, the needle procedure is quite painful, and therefore it isn't performed very often.

Magnetic resonance imaging

Magnetic resonance imaging (MRI) uses a magnet and radio waves to create detailed, layered (cross-sectional) images of body tissues — in this case, the anal sphincter muscles and surrounding area. MRI is more expensive than are other tests; therefore, its cost needs to be weighed against the advantages it offers.

For a traditional MRI, you lie very still on a table that's rolled into the opening of a large, tunnel-shaped magnet. Some MRI machines have an open scanner that doesn't require you to be in an enclosed space.

Before the test, a contrast dye will be given to you in a vein (intravenously). The dye shows the response of body tissues to being in a magnetic field and allows the MRI machine to create images of the inside of the body. To get a clearer picture of your anal sphincters, a slim coil or tube may be inserted in your rectum.

A newer form of MRI called dynamic MRI is very valuable in evaluating problems with the pelvic floor, rectum and anus. Dynamic MRI creates a real-time image of your pelvic floor as you contract your pelvic floor muscles and move your bowels, allowing the doctor to see any abnormalities that occur as you defecate.

For the test, your rectum is filled with ultrasound gel. While you're lying in the MRI machine, you pass the gel out as if it were stool. The machine creates a series of images of the defecation process.

Dynamic MRI is useful for identifying anal sphincter problems, pelvic floor problems, such as rectal prolapse, and rectoceles.

Defecography

This test shows how much and how well your rectum can hold stool and how well your rectum works during defecation. Like dynamic MRI, it provides a visual picture of the dynamics of defecation. Defecography may be useful for evaluating suspected rectal prolapse or other problems or if you're having trouble completely emptying your rectum.

For the procedure, your doctor inserts a small amount of barium paste into your rectum. Barium coats the walls of your rectum and makes it visible on X-rays. You sit on a specially designed seat similar to a toilet. Motion in your pelvic floor can be recorded on video or X-rays as you rest, cough, squeeze and strain to pass the barium out of your rectum.

TEST RESULTS

The results of your tests, along with your symptoms and history, help your doctor reach a diagnosis and develop an appropriate treatment plan. The test results may also provide your doctor with much more information about the appearance and function of your bowels.

As your doctor lays out your treatment plan, it's important that the two of you discuss your test results and treatment options. The best treatment plan is generally one in which you and your doctor have explored your options together and reached a consensus based on your particular circumstances and wants and your doctor's knowledge and experience.

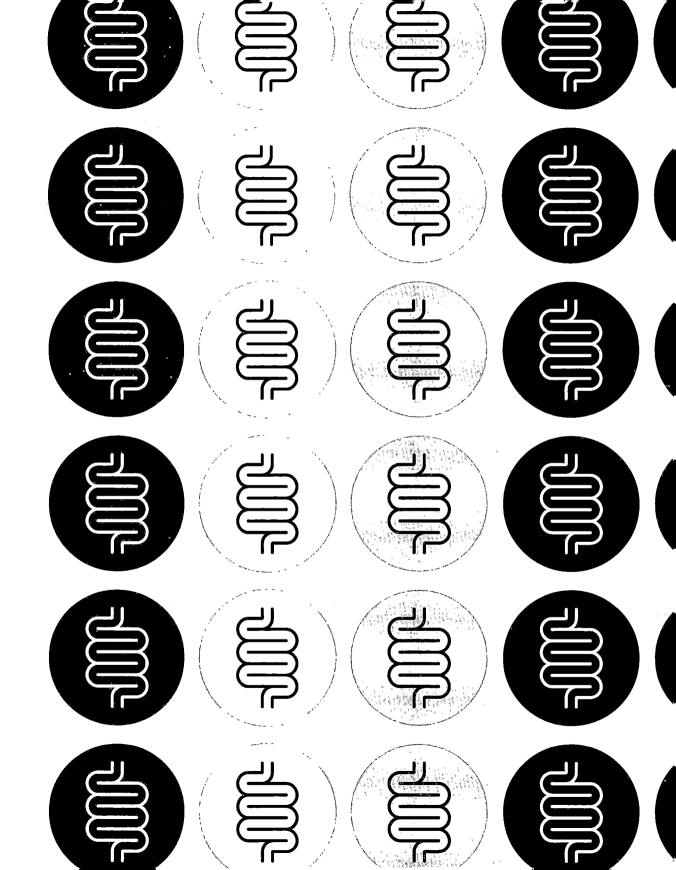

11

Treating fecal incontinence

Seeking help for fecal incontinence is an important first step in managing the condition. Acknowledging the problem and working with a sympathetic, supportive doctor can ease some of the feelings of isolation, embarrassment and depression that many people with fecal incontinence experience.

Fortunately, effective treatments are available for fecal incontinence. Treatment usually can help restore bowel control or at least substantially reduce the severity of your symptoms. An important goal of treatment is to improve your quality of life. Various coping strategies can make living with fecal incontinence easier.

The treatment you will receive depends on the cause of your incontinence and

how severe it is. Treatment normally starts with nonsurgical options. These are sometimes referred to as conservative, or behavioral, therapies and may include changing your diet, regulating your bowel habits and using biofeedback. In some cases, inserts or medication may be an option.

For many people, the simplest treatments provide substantial relief. If conservative approaches don't work, your doctor may recommend surgery.

Because incontinence often results from more than one cause, more than one form of treatment may be needed to achieve successful bowel control. Your doctor also may need to address certain medical conditions that may be contributing to your incontinence. These may include diseases or disorders such as impacted stool, dementia, neurological problems, inflammatory bowel disease and lactose intolerance.

CONSERVATIVE TREATMENTS

Treating fecal incontinence often begins with steps to modify your behavior and your habits. These approaches may be all that's necessary to bring incontinence under control, or they may be combined with other treatments.

Almost everyone can gain some benefit from conservative treatments. Studies suggest they not only help with incontinence but also improve quality of life, psychological well-being and anal sphincter function. Conservative treatments also may cause you to feel more in control and more confident that you can deal with incontinence episodes should they occur.

Diet

Diet has a major effect on bowel function. What you eat and drink affects the consistency of your stool and how quickly it passes through your digestive system. Changes to your diet can improve your bowel movements and make them more predictable.

Your doctor will help you find a diet that helps you gain good stool consistency. You'll also want to avoid foods that irritate your digestive system. Following are some dietary factors that may affect your bowel control.

Fiber

Foods that are high in fiber can help improve the consistency of stool, making it softer, bulkier and more formed. A soft, bulky stool is easier to pass than a hard, small stool. Formed stool is also less likely to leak out than is stool that's more watery.

A fiber-rich diet promotes more-frequent and regular bowel movements, and it can help control both constipation and diarrhea.

Fiber, also known as roughage or bulk, includes all parts of plant foods that your body can't digest or absorb. It's found mainly in fruits, vegetables, whole grains and legumes. Other sources of dietary fiber are listed on pages 156-157.

There are two types of fiber, soluble and insoluble. Insoluble fiber doesn't dissolve in water. It moves through your digestive system quickly, making the stool bulkier. Insoluble fiber is found in bananas, brown rice, tapioca, whole-grain bread, potatoes, applesauce, cheese, yogurt, pasta and oatmeal.

Soluble fiber dissolves in water to form a soft, gel-like material in the intestines. This type of fiber is found in oat bran, beans, barley, nuts, seeds, lentils, peas, apples, citrus fruits and carrots.

So how much fiber should you eat? Experts recommend approximately 20 to 40 grams a day. You generally need less as you age. Women age 51 and older should aim for approximately 20 grams a day,

CONTROLLING GAS

Even as your bowel control improves, you'll still pass gas. Everyone has gas in his or her digestive tracts. Dietary changes can help control excessive gas.

Gas in the digestive tract comes from two main sources — swallowed air and the breakdown of undigested food in the large intestine. Most foods that contain carbohydrates can cause gas. Gas-producing foods include:
- Beans
- Some vegetables, such as asparagus, broccoli, cabbage, Brussels sprouts, cauliflower, cucumbers, green peppers, onions and radishes
- Some fruits, such as apples, peaches and pears
- Whole grains and bran
- Carbonated drinks
- Milk and milk products
- Packaged foods made with lactose, such as bread, cereal and salad dressing
- Foods with sorbitol, such as sugar-free candies and gums

Foods more likely to form odorous gas include asparagus, beans, cabbage, coffee, cucumbers, dairy products, eggs, garlic, nuts, onions and radishes.

If gas is a problem, keep a food diary for a week or so to identify what foods may cause gas or affect its odor. Many of the foods that cause gas, such as fruits, vegetables and whole grains, are important parts of a healthy diet, so the solution isn't to cut them out altogether. Experiment to find out how much of the offending foods you can handle.

Several over-the-counter medications can help reduce symptoms. These include antacids with simethicone, activated charcoal tablets and alpha-galactosidase (Beano). If you have problems with milk and other dairy products, the enzyme lactase can help you digest lactose, the sugar in milk. Lactase is available in liquid and tablet form, or you can buy lactose-reduced milk and other products.

---

and men age 51 and older should get closer to 30 grams daily.

Be aware that adding too much fiber to your diet at once can cause bloating, gas or diarrhea. Too much insoluble fiber also can contribute to diarrhea. If eating more fiber seems to make your diarrhea worse, cut back to two servings each a day of fruits and vegetables. Removing the skins and the seeds from your food also can help reduce symptoms.

Here's a look at the fiber content of some common foods. Read nutrition labels to find out how much fiber is in your favorite foods.

	Serving size	Total fiber (grams)
Fruits		
Pear	1 medium	5.5
Apple, with skin	1 medium	4.4
Raspberries	½ cup	4.0
Blueberries	1 cup	3.6
Peaches, dried	3 halves	3.2
Orange	1 medium	3.1
Strawberries	1 cup	3.0
Apricots, dried	10 halves	2.6
Figs, dried	2 medium	1.6
Raisins	1½-ounce box	1.6
Grains, cereals and pastas		
Spaghetti, whole-grain	1 cup	9.1
Bran flakes cereal	1 cup	7.8
Oatmeal, old-fashioned	½ cup	4.0
Bread, whole-wheat	1 slice	2.2
Bread, rye	1 slice	1.9
Bread, multigrain	1 slice	1.9
Bread, cracked wheat	1 slice	1.1

	Serving size	Total fiber (grams)
Legumes, nuts and seeds		
Navy beans, cooked	1 cup	19.1
Black beans, cooked	1 cup	15.0
Lentils, cooked	1 cup	14.2
Peanuts, roasted, unshelled	1 cup	13.7
Lima beans, cooked	1 cup	12.6
Sunflower seed kernels	½ cup	6.0
Cashews	1 cup	3.9
Almonds	23 nuts	3.5
Pistachio nuts	49 nuts	3.0

	Serving size	Total fiber (grams)
Vegetables		
Artichoke hearts, cooked	1 cup	9.6
Peas	1 cup	8.2
Spinach, chopped, cooked	1 cup	7.6
Turnip greens, boiled	1 cup	5.0
Brussels sprouts, cooked	1 cup	4.1
Potato, baked with skin	1 medium	3.6
Corn	1 cup	2.9
Broccoli	1 cup	2.3
Carrot	1 medium	1.7
Popcorn, microwaved	1 cup	1.1
Tomato paste	2 tablespoons	1.0

Source: FoodData Central. U.S. Department of Agriculture, Agriculture Research Service. https://fdc.nal.usda.gov

As you increase your fiber intake, it's important to drink plenty of water. Fiber works best when it absorbs water. Without enough fluids, stool becomes hard, and this can lead to constipation.

You can also boost your fiber intake with supplements such as Metamucil, Citrucel and FiberCon, which help move water into the bowel and propel stool toward the rectum. Fiber supplements can increase stool volume and reduce watery stools.

Supplements may be helpful for some people, but they can worsen diarrhea or incontinence in others. Supplements also don't provide the vitamins, minerals and other nutrients found in high-fiber foods. Talk to your doctor about use of fiber supplements.

Also keep in mind that increasing fiber intake isn't helpful for everyone. Older adults who are inactive may have more problems with incontinence if they eat a high-fiber diet. For people with constipation resulting from a slowed digestive system, too much fiber can cause bloating and abdominal pain.

Fluids

To prevent dehydration and keep your stools soft and formed, drink plenty of water and other liquids. Fluids help foods move through the digestive system and keep you from getting constipated.

Try to consume about 60 ounces of fluids daily — approximately eight 8-ounce glasses of fluid (the 8x8 rule). Avoid caffeine-containing beverages, alcohol, milk and carbonated drinks if you find that they contribute to diarrhea.

If you're prone to diarrhea or you often have a feeling of urgency to use the toilet, you can slow the digestive process by drinking fluids at different times than when you eat. For example, have a glass of water, soda or other beverage an hour or more before or after a meal, and drink less with your meals.

Caffeine

Coffee and other beverages and foods that contain caffeine can act as laxatives, causing diarrhea or an urgent need to use the toilet. Reducing how much caffeine you consume each day, especially after meals, may help lessen diarrhea and the sense of urgency you experience when you need to go to the bathroom.

A list of foods and beverages that may worsen fecal incontinence appears on page 183.

Meal portions and timing

For some people, large meals promote bowel contractions that can lead to diarrhea. You can avoid this by eating several smaller meals throughout the day rather than three large ones.

In general, eating at regular times each day and eating well-balanced meals will help with bowel regularity.

Medications

Some medications can contribute to fecal incontinence. Tell your doctor about any medications and vitamin and mineral supplements that you take. Your doctor may suggest a change in your medications if he or she suspects they may be causing diarrhea, constipation or incontinence. A list of medications that can contribute to fecal incontinence or make it worse appears on page 186.

Bowel training

Establishing regular bowel habits is a simple approach that can make a big difference in managing incontinence. Bowel training can help some people relearn how to control their bowels. It can also help restore muscle strength if your fecal incontinence stems from a lack of anal sphincter control or from decreased awareness of the urge to defecate.

A program of bowel training involves several steps and strategies aimed at producing regular bowel movements. In some cases, bowel training means going to the toilet at set times of the day. In other instances, the training involves exercise therapy.

Some people achieve bowel control by making a conscious effort to have bowel movements at specific times during the day, such as after a meal. Having some predictability regarding your bowel movements can give you some confidence that you won't need to rush to the bathroom unexpectedly.

Regular bowel movements also may reduce your risk of constipation, which can lead to fecal incontinence.

Before you start a bowel training program, your doctor will want to make sure you don't have fecal impaction. The impacted stool must be removed before bowel training can work.

Here are some suggestions on how to get your digestive system on a regular bathroom schedule:

- *Establish a set time for daily bowel movements.* Choose times that are convenient for you, keeping in mind your daily schedule and your past patterns of elimination. The best time for a bowel movement generally is 20 to 30 minutes after a meal because eating stimulates bowel activity and your rectum is likely to be full, even if you don't feel a need to go. The goal is to establish a routine — moving your bowels at the same time each day.
- *Practice.* If you have constipation or irritable bowel syndrome, it may take some time before you're able to go "on demand." Try sitting on the toilet for a few minutes, even if you don't feel like you need to go or if you don't actually have a bowel movement. With practice your bowels may be stimulated to work more effectively. However, sitting too long may contribute to the development of hemorrhoids. If you're unsuccessful after a few minutes, it's usually better to get up and walk around a bit, then try again.
- *Drink warm fluids.* Some people find it helpful to drink hot tea or warm prune juice to stimulate a bowel movement.

If you have a mass of hard stool in your rectum (impacted stool), the first line of treatment is to remove it. If taking laxatives or using enemas doesn't help you pass the mass, your doctor may have to assist in removing it. To do so, a doctor inserts one or two fingers into your rectum and breaks the impacted stool into fragments that you can then expel.

After the impacted stool is expelled, your doctor may suggest a number of steps to prevent constipation, such as increasing your intake of fiber and fluids and becoming more physically active. Other ways to prevent constipation and impacted stool include use of mild laxatives, stool softeners, enemas and suppositories. Consult your doctor regarding the product you should use.

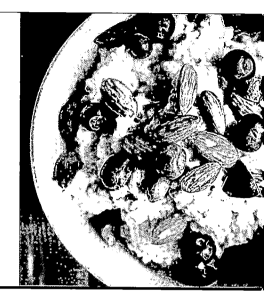

- **Try stimulation.** Your doctor may recommend that you try stimulating a bowel movement by inserting a lubricated finger into your anus. Move your finger in a circular motion until the sphincter muscle relaxes. It might take a few minutes.
- **Experiment with suppositories, enemas, laxatives or a combination.** They can stimulate a bowel movement but should only be used with your doctor's advice. It's best to use the least stimulation that's effective.
- **Relax.** Try to relax when you're on the toilet and assume a posture that's conducive to defecating. Avoid straining.

Persistence and consistency are the keys to success. It may take a while to form a regular pattern. Try not to get frustrated and give up if it doesn't happen right away. Most people can achieve regular

bowel movements within a few weeks of starting a bowel training program.

Tailor bowel training to your individual situation. For example, if you have a rectal prolapse or rectocele, your focus may be on reducing the number of attempts to have a bowel movement and to avoid excessive straining. In this situation, you might be advised to attempt to have a bowel movement no more than three times a day.

Pelvic floor muscle exercises

No matter what the cause of your fecal incontinence, your doctor may recommend exercises (Kegel exercises) to strengthen your pelvic floor, sphincter and rectal muscles. These exercises can be combined with other treatments and

One way to keep your bowels moving is to keep your body moving. Regular physical exercise stimulates intestinal muscle activity, helping to move food waste through your intestines. Lack of physical activity is a common cause of constipation in older adults and people whose mobility is limited because of a stroke, a spinal injury or another medical condition.

Staying physically active can help promote regular bowel movements and help prevent constipation. But if you are prone to diarrhea or have trouble holding in stool, brisk physical activity — particularly after meals or soon after waking up in the morning — may lead to incontinence.

Use a bowel symptom diary (see page 184) to chart whether and when exercise triggers an incontinence episode. You may need to exercise at a different time of day or choose more-moderate activities.

---

are used as part of biofeedback treatment. Pelvic floor muscle training is described in detail, beginning on page 179.

Biofeedback

Biofeedback is a way to receive visual, audio or verbal feedback about a body function you normally don't perceive, such as muscle activity. Biofeedback may be used to help strengthen and coordinate the muscles involved in holding in stool. It can also improve your ability to sense the presence of stool in your rectum.

Many people with fecal incontinence gain at least some benefit from biofeedback. The technique may be useful if your incontinence is due to weak sphincter muscles, impaired rectal sensation, chronic constipation or nerve damage from diabetes, childbirth or surgery. People with severe fecal incontinence or underlying neurological diseases may be less likely to benefit. In addition, biofeedback may not be useful for individuals with no or very limited rectal sensation.

Because biofeedback is safe and effective, it's often recommended before considering surgery. Whether biofeedback will work for you depends on the cause of your incontinence and the severity of the muscle or nerve damage. The success of this approach also depends on your own motivation and on the biofeedback therapist's experience and expertise.

Techniques

One biofeedback technique involves inserting a pressure-sensitive probe into your anal canal. The probe registers the strength and activity of your anal sphincter muscle as it contracts around the probe. The person performing the test will teach you how to squeeze your anal muscles around the probe.

You can practice sphincter contractions at home and learn to strengthen the sphincter muscles by viewing the scale's readout or by listening to the audio responses.

Biofeedback helps ensure that you're doing the exercises correctly and it indicates whether your muscles are getting stronger.

Another biofeedback technique uses manometry equipment to vary the pressure in your rectum. (For more information on manometry, see page 146). In this procedure, a probe with a deflated balloon is inserted into your rectum. The practitioner then inflates the balloon to various levels, training you to detect smaller amounts of stool in your rectum through the use of feedback. Yet another technique uses three balloons and teaches you to respond to sensation in your rectum by immediately and forcefully squeezing your anal sphincter muscle.

Results

A typical biofeedback program requires four to six sessions. Sometimes, one session is all you need. Most people see an improvement in symptoms after three sessions.

For the best results, it's important that you feel comfortable with your biofeedback therapist. You may have the treatment at a biofeedback clinic, at your doctor's office or at the office of a therapist trained in biofeedback. He or she will likely begin by asking a number of questions about your bowel habits and history. The therapist can also provide support, advice and education about your bowel habits.

In addition to training you to use your sphincter muscles, the therapist may also teach you techniques for proper defecation, as well as relaxation techniques. This is because many people with fecal incontinence become anxious when they feel the urge to go.

PRODUCTS AND DEVICES

Various products and devices can help reduce the severity and frequency of fecal incontinence. These items may be used to help manage your condition or to keep you dry while waiting for other treatments to take effect.

Vaginal insert

This newer device, also sometimes referred to as an inflatable vaginal balloon, is inserted into the female vagina in the same location as a tampon or a diaphragm. Called Eclipse, the insert is ring-shaped and it contains an inflatable balloon and an attached tube that extends outside the vagina. A small, hand-held pump that you attach to the extending tube is used to inflate and deflate the balloon.

When the balloon is inflated, it places pressure on the adjacent rectal area (see the illustration at right below) preventing stool from passing and decreasing episodes of fecal incontinence. When you're ready to have a bowel movement, you deflate the balloon (see illustration at left). After passage of stool, you inflate the balloon again until your next bowel movement.

The device is fitted for each individual, and it can be inserted or removed at any time. It's recommended that you remove it weekly for cleaning. Your doctor will provide instructions on how to insert, remove and clean the device. You'll also be instructed on how to inflate and deflate the balloon.

Women interested in the device are typically given an insert to use for a short trial period to see how well it works and to make sure it fits comfortably. In case of sizing issues, alterations can be made.

If you're satisfied with the performance of the insert and your quality of life, your doctor will prescribe the device for you. The Food and Drug Administration has determined that Eclipse needs to be replaced yearly. Early studies indicate most women who've tried the insert have found it to be comfortable and effective.

MEDICATIONS

Medications may be part of your treatment plan for fecal incontinence if you have loose, watery stools or diarrhea, or if chronic constipation is causing your fecal

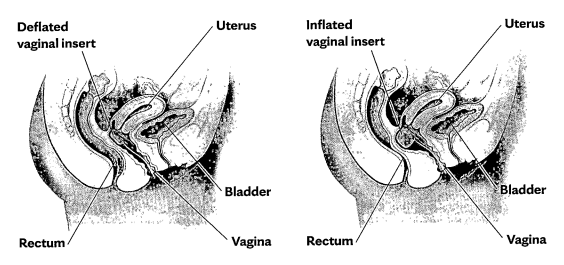

To prevent leakage, a balloon attached to the insert is inflated, placing pressure on the rectum (right). When it's time for a bowel movement, it's deflated (left).

incontinence. Your doctor will try to identify and treat the underlying disorder that's causing the diarrhea or constipation. If a disorder can't be found or corrected, you may be given a medication to relieve your symptoms and restore bowel control.

Diarrhea medications

As a first step in treating diarrhea or loose stools, your doctor may recommend that you include more high-fiber foods in your diet or that you take an over-the-counter anti-diarrheal agent. Fiber supplements such as Metamucil and Citrucel also can help because they make stools bulkier and less fluid.

The anti-diarrheal drug most commonly used in treating fecal incontinence is loperamide (Imodium A-D), which is available without a prescription. Loperamide slows down bowel activity, reducing stool frequency and making stools more formed. The drug has the added benefit of increasing rectal and anal sensitivity, which also improves bowel control. Taking loperamide before going out for a meal or social event may help you avoid an incontinent episode in public.

Your doctor can help you determine the proper dose of loperamide. Side effects are generally mild but may include constipation, abdominal cramping, dry mouth and nausea.

Other anti-diarrheal medications sometimes used to treat fecal incontinence include products containing diphenoxy-late (Lomotil), difenoxin (Motofen) and alosetron (Lotronex). Some of these medications are available without a prescription.

Constipation medications

If chronic constipation is causing your incontinence, your doctor may recommend the temporary use of mild laxatives, such as milk of magnesia, to help restore normal bowel movements. To prevent stool impaction, your doctor may recommend a fiber supplement such as Metamucil, Citrucel or FiberCon, or a laxative such as MiraLax.

The prescription medication lubiprostone (Amitiza) may be used as a short-term treatment for women with irritable bowel syndrome who have constipation as their main bowel problem, or for women under age 65 who have chronic constipation.

Other medications

There currently aren't any medications specifically approved for the treatment of fecal incontinence. Drugs used to treat inflammatory bowel disease are sometimes used to control fecal incontinence. If you have a question about medications, talk with your doctor.

COPING STRATEGIES

It can take time for fecal incontinence therapies to work, and sometimes the condition can't be completely corrected.

TREATING DOUBLE INCONTINENCE

Many people experience both urinary and fecal incontinence, also known as double incontinence. The two conditions can stem from many of the same causes, including muscle and nerve damage from childbirth, years of straining to have bowel movements, muscular weakness with aging, and diseases that cause nerve damage.

If you have combined urinary and fecal incontinence, you may need to see more than one doctor or find someone who has experience in both areas. You might see a specialist in a female pelvic medicine and reconstructive surgery or a gynecologist, urologist, colorectal surgeon, or gastroenterologist.

Treatment for double incontinence typically begins with behavioral therapies, including pelvic floor muscle exercises, bladder and bowel training, and biofeedback. Surgery may be recommended to repair both an anal sphincter defect and pelvic floor problems. Sacral nerve stimulation (see page 167) is sometimes recommended for people with both fecal and urinary urge incontinence.

For these reasons, you may not be able to avoid having an occasional accident. Having a plan for these times helps lessen feelings of fear, embarrassment, anger, isolation, humiliation and loneliness.

Fear of having an accident may keep you from wanting to go out in public, go to work or attend social events. To help overcome this fear, consider these practical tips:

- Use the toilet before heading out.
- Carry cleanup supplies and a change of clothing.
- If you think an episode is likely while you're out, wear pads or disposable undergarments.
- Locate public restrooms before you need to use them.

- Be flexible. If you don't feel comfortable leaving the house on a particular day, change the activity to another day.

Self-care products

There are a variety of products such as absorbent pads and disposable underwear that can help you better manage incontinence.

Understandably, it can be difficult to accept that you need to use such items, but don't let that keep you from taking advantage of products that can help. You can purchase incontinence products at drugstores, supermarkets, medical supply stores or online.

If you care for someone with fecal incontinence, try to be supportive and not critical. Consider these tips:
• Make regular trips to the bathroom with your loved one to help him or her avoid an accident.
• Make sure clothing is easy to open or remove.
• Place a portable toilet (commode) near the bed.
• Use washable cushions or slipcovers.
• Use absorbent undergarments and washable bed pads.
• Clean the skin around the person's anal area immediately after an incontinent episode. Follow the suggestions on this page for keeping the anal area clean and dry.

If you use pads or adult diapers, be sure that they have an absorbent wicking layer on top. Products with this layer protect your skin by pulling stool and moisture away from skin and into the pad.

Relieving anal discomfort

The skin around your anus is delicate and sensitive. Diarrhea, constipation or contact between stool and skin can cause pain or itching. Consider the following practices to relieve anal discomfort and eliminate possible odor.
• Gently wash the area around your anus with plain water after each bowel movement, either by using wet toilet paper, showering or soaking in a bath. Soap can dry skin, worsening irritation. Avoid rubbing with dry toilet paper. Pre-moistened, alcohol-free towelettes are a good choice for cleaning the area.
• Allow the area to air-dry after washing. If you don't have time, gently pat the area dry with clean toilet paper or a clean washcloth. A hair dryer may help, but be sure it's set on the cool setting.
• Apply a moisture-barrier cream to keep irritated skin from direct contact with stool. Ask your doctor to recommend a product. Be sure the area is clean before applying the cream. You can also try nonmedicated talcum powder or cornstarch to relieve anal discomfort.
• Wear cotton underwear and loose clothing. Tight clothing can restrict airflow and worsen anal problems. Change soiled underwear right away.
• If it helps you feel more comfortable, consider using a deodorizing body wash or spray.

SURGERY AND OTHER THERAPIES

Most people with fecal incontinence don't need surgery. But if other treatments aren't successful and the incontinence remains severe and disabling, surgical options may be considered. Surgery may be helpful for people whose incontinence is caused by damage to the pelvic floor, anal canal or anal sphincter, perhaps from a tear during childbirth, a fracture or a past operation.

Various surgical procedures may be performed. They range from minor repair of damaged tissues to complex surgeries. Sometimes a combination of procedures may be used. Surgery isn't free of complications, but it's often effective.

Sacral nerve stimulation

A newer treatment for fecal incontinence involves electrical stimulation of the sacral nerves. These are the nerves that run from your spinal cord to the muscles in your pelvis. The sacral nerves regulate the sensation and strength of your rectal and anal sphincter muscles.

Direct electrical stimulation of the sacral nerves was first shown to be effective in treating urinary incontinence. Later studies found that the procedure may also help fecal incontinence. This treatment may be recommended if behavior therapy and medications have failed to improve fecal incontinence, or for people who are still experiencing incontinence after surgery to repair the anal sphincter.

Sacral nerve stimulation is generally done in an operating room at a hospital or outpatient clinic. You'll receive a medication for sedation, as well as a local anesthetic in the involved area — on your backside, below your waist and above where you sit.

The surgery is done in stages. First the doctor uses an X-ray device to identify the places in the triangular bone in the middle of your pelvis (sacrum) where the sacral nerves are located. A needle is inserted into the sacral nerves that control the bowel, bladder and pelvic floor. The needle is connected to an external device that generates electrical pulses that stimulate the nerves. The doctor checks muscle and sensory responses to this electrical stimulation.

Once the proper responses have been noted, the permanent wire (lead) is placed next to the sacral nerve. The lead is tunneled under the skin and connected to another lead that passes outside the skin. During this initial phase, electrical stimulation is controlled through a small battery-powered unit that you carry. If your incontinence and quality of life improve with electrical stimulation, you may then return and have the external wire removed and an implantable, programmable battery unit placed under the skin (see page 89).

The battery unit (generator) is placed in your upper buttocks and connected to the permanent wire. It produces electrical impulses that stimulate the sacral nerves, helping you regain continence. The generator has an external control unit that allows you to adjust the programming. Appointments with your doctor every four to six months are recommended to make sure the device is programmed correctly.

You can choose between a rechargeable battery or a nonrechargeable battery to be used in the generator. Both batteries and their leads are compatible with magnetic resonance imaging (MRI). The advantage of the rechargeable battery is that it's smaller. It needs to be charged once a week, taking about 20 minutes. Discuss with your doctor which option may be best for you.

Sacral nerve stimulation is much less invasive than are other surgical approaches and has other advantages as well. The procedure carries low risks of serious complications and won't worsen symptoms or cause nerve damage.

Sphincteroplasty

Sphincteroplasty is surgery to repair a damaged anal sphincter. The operation is effective for people who have a single site of injury in the anal sphincter, such as a tear that occurred during vaginal delivery. A tear or interruption in the ring of muscle that makes up the external anal sphincter can prevent it from closing tightly enough to hold stool in.

During a sphincteroplasty, the surgeon identifies the injured area of muscle and frees its edges from the surrounding tissue. The muscle edges are then brought back and sewn together in an overlapping fashion to create a complete ring of muscle, restoring the anus to its proper shape. This helps tighten the sphincter.

You'll likely be in the hospital for several days, and it may be a month or more before you return to your usual activities.

During the recovery period, you may experience discomfort, bruising and swelling at the surgical site. It's important to carefully follow the instructions regarding cleaning and caring for the wound to avoid infections. The first few days after surgery you'll likely need to use a urinary catheter.

About two-thirds of people who have the operation benefit from the procedure. However, long-term success rates are lower, particularly when nerve injury is involved. About half the people who have this surgery experience some degree of incontinence again or have to deal with certain lifestyle restrictions. Some require further surgery.

Mayo Clinic generally recommends this procedure only when done very shortly after the initial injury. Otherwise, incontinence tends to recur a year or two after the operation. In women who sustain sphincter injury during delivery and who wish to have more children, it may be best to delay the repair until they finish their families or plan for future children to be delivered via cesarean section (C-section).

Even when surgery is successful, you still might not have complete bowel control. Your doctor may suggest biofeedback treatment after surgery to help you gain better control of your anal sphincter.

Radiofrequency therapy

Radiofrequency therapy, known as the Secca procedure, involves delivering temperature-controlled radiofrequency energy to the wall of the anal canal. A probe inserted into the anus directs controlled amounts of heat energy into the anal wall. The radiofrequency energy creates mild injury to the sphincter muscles in the form of thermal lesions, while preserving muscle integrity.

The goal of the treatment is to create muscle changes to improve muscle tone. Over time, as the thermal lesions heal, the tissue contracts and the muscles become thicker, improving symptoms of incontinence. The procedure is minimally invasive and is generally performed under local anesthesia and sedation. A drawback of the procedure, however, is that it isn't always covered by insurance.

Other procedures

Depending on the cause of your incontinence and the severity of your symptoms, other procedures may be considered.

Treatment of associated conditions

Rectal prolapse is a condition in which a portion of your rectum protrudes through your anus and weakens the anal sphincter. In certain circumstances, such as with chronic constipation and straining, the ligaments in the rectum can become stretched and lose their ability to hold stool in place.

Surgical correction of the rectal prolapse, along with sphincter muscle repair, may provide treatment for fecal incontinence. Sometimes, though, incontinence can worsen after prolapse repair.

In women, protrusion of the rectum into the vagina (rectocele) can cause problems that may need to be corrected surgically (see illustration below).

Hemorrhoids also may pose a problem. Prolapsed internal hemorrhoids can cause seepage of mucus, giving the sensation of constant moisture in the anal

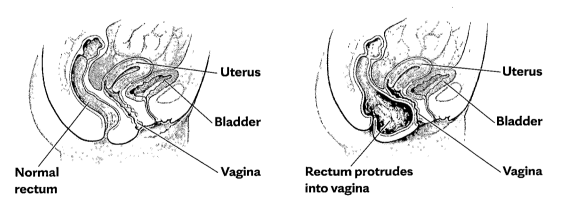

Rectocele is a hernial protrusion of part of the rectum into the vagina. Weakened pelvic floor muscles can lead to rectocele and fecal incontinence.

area. Hemorrhoids may be near the upper part or beginning of the anal canal (internal hemorrhoids) or at the lower portion or anal opening (external hemorrhoids).

Severe hemorrhoids can be treated with a surgical procedure (hemorrhoidectomy) to remove the hemorrhoidal tissue. However, overaggressive hemorrhoidectomy can lead to fecal incontinence.

Bulking agents

Injections of materials into tissue located beneath the anal lining may help build tissue in the area surrounding the internal anal sphincter. By growing (bulking) the surrounding tissue, the opening of the anus narrows, stopping or limiting leakage of stool. Control of the anal sphincter muscles also may improve.

A bulking agent called Solesta can help with fecal incontinence. Solesta contains microbeads within a gel made up of dextranomer and sodium hyaluronate. The substance is injected into the anal canal in four locations to bulk up the canal. The procedure is done on an outpatient basis, and it may be repeated if the first injections aren't effective.

Other types of materials that add bulk to anal tissues are being studied, but are not yet available for clinical use.

The downside of most bulking agents is that they lose their effectiveness over time and repeat injections are usually needed. And similar to radiofrequency

therapy, bulking agents may not be covered by insurance.

Colostomy

As a last resort, colostomy surgery may be the most definitive way to correct fecal incontinence, particularly in older adults. In a colostomy, a surgeon attaches the end of the large intestine to an opening in the abdomen. A collection device is attached to this opening to collect the stool.

A colostomy can often be performed with a minimally invasive surgical procedure that requires a few small incisions. The colostomy device isn't visible when you're dressed, and it controls odor very effectively. For many people, a colostomy offers a more socially acceptable alternative to severe, uncontrolled fecal incontinence.

FUTURE CARE

Researchers are working on an artificial bowel sphincter that would operate on a similar concept as the artificial sphincter used to treat urinary incontinence (see page 90).

Until such a product becomes available, most people can find some relief from the options discussed in this chapter. With the help of a sensitive, knowledgeable doctor and by undergoing the right diagnostic tests, you can receive treatment that provides good results and improves your quality of life.

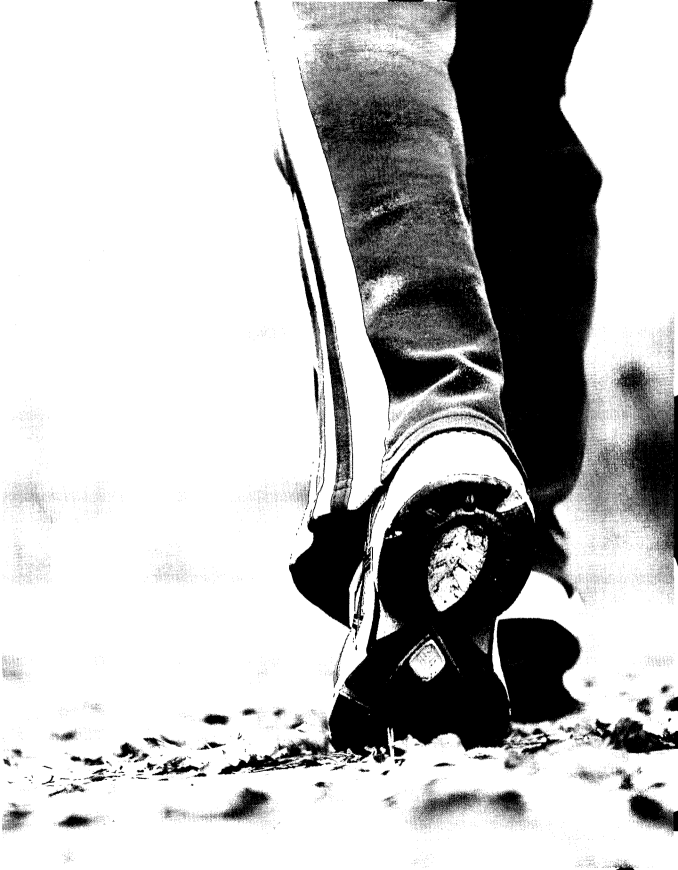

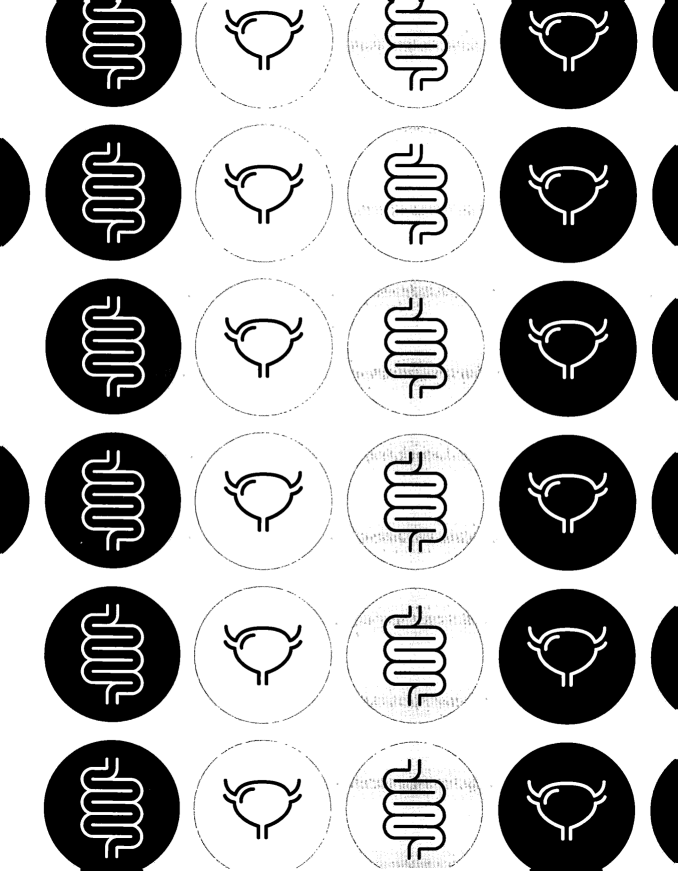

Appendix

The following pages provide helpful information to assist you in determining if you have urinary or fecal incontinence, and how to manage the condition. You'll find lists of foods, beverages and medications that may play a role in your incontinence, along with suggestions on things you can do to reduce signs and symptoms.

We begin with information specific to urinary incontinence, followed by information pertinent to fecal incontinence. On the last page are questions to help you find the right doctor for your condition.

BLADDER DIARY

A bladder diary is a detailed, day-to-day account of your symptoms and other information related to your urinary habits. A sample bladder diary is found on pages 174-175. You record what and how much you drink, when you urinate, the amount of urine you produce, whether you had an urge to urinate, and the number of incontinence episodes. To measure your urine, your doctor may give you a device that fits over your toilet rim with markings similar to a measuring cup. A simpler alternative is to describe the quantity in more general terms, such as small, medium or large.

Keep a bladder diary for two to seven consecutive days and nights. You want it to represent your normal day. Don't keep a diary during vacations or other changes in routine. If you're female, don't start the diary during your menstrual period, when you may need to visit the bathroom more often.

	Fluids You Drank (Intake)		Urinated in the Toilet (Output)	
Time *(hh:mm)*	Amount	Type	Time *(hh:mm)*	Amount
	oz			oz
	oz			oz
	oz			oz
	oz			oz
	oz			oz
	oz			oz
	oz			oz
	oz			oz
	oz			oz
	oz			oz
	oz			oz
	oz			oz
	oz			oz
	oz			oz
	oz			oz
	oz			oz
	oz			oz
	oz			oz
	oz			oz
	oz			oz
	oz			oz
Total Daily Intake	**oz**		**Total Daily Output**	**oz**

Accidental Urine Leakage

Time *(hh:mm)*	Amount	Urge Yes	No	Activity
	oz	☐	☐	
	oz	☐	☐	
	oz	☐	☐	
	oz	☐	☐	
	oz	☐	☐	
	oz	☐	☐	
	oz	☐	☐	
	oz	☐	☐	
	oz	☐	☐	
	oz	☐	☐	
	oz	☐	☐	
	oz	☐	☐	
	oz	☐	☐	
	oz	☐	☐	
	oz	☐	☐	
	oz	☐	☐	
	oz	☐	☐	
	oz	☐	☐	

How many times did you urinate in 24 hours?	
Number and type of pads used during the day:	
Number and type of pads used during the night:	

DIETARY RESTRICTIONS

Some of the things that you eat or drink can irritate your bladder and aggravate signs and symptoms of incontinence. By keeping a diary of what you eat and drink and your signs and symptoms, you may begin to see a connection between certain foods and beverages and episodes of incontinence.

If you identify a food or beverage that seems to be causing problems, try reducing or eliminating that item from your diet for a week or two. If your signs and symptoms improve, consider avoiding the item permanently or at least reducing how much of it you consume.

Bladder irritants

The following list includes foods and beverages that can lead to bladder irritability. Remember that it's not necessary to completely cut out all of the items listed here. But if one or more of these items seem to be causing you problems, you may want to significantly reduce how much you consume, or avoid the items altogether.

Carbonated beverages
- Soda
- Sparkling water

Alcohol
- Beer
- Liquor
- Wine, wine coolers

Caffeine
- Coffee
- Tea
- Chocolate
- Some medications
- Some supplements

Citrus fruits and juices
- Orange
- Grapefruit
- Lemon
- Lime
- Mango
- Pineapple
- Vitamin C supplements

Tomatoes and tomato-based foods
- Tomato juice
- Tomato sauce
- Barbecue sauce
- Chili

Onions and spicy foods
- Foods that use chili peppers or other pungent spices (Mexican, Thai, Indian, Cajun)

Foods containing vinegar
- Pickled foods
- Dressings
- Some condiments

Products containing aspartame and saccharin
- Diet soda
- Sugar-free ice cream
- Sugar-fee cocoa mix
- Sugarless candy
- Some vitamins, supplements and medications

SAMPLE FOOD AND BEVERAGE DIARY

| Time (hh:mm) | Food or beverage | How much | Problem signs or symptoms | | |
			Yes	No	When
7:30 a.m.	coffee	2 cups	■	☐	8:30 a.m.
			☐	☐	
			☐	☐	
			☐	☐	
			☐	☐	
			☐	☐	
			☐	☐	
			☐	☐	
			☐	☐	
			☐	☐	
			☐	☐	
			☐	☐	
			☐	☐	
			☐	☐	
			☐	☐	
			☐	☐	
			☐	☐	
			☐	☐	
			☐	☐	
			☐	☐	

PROBLEM MEDICATIONS

Medications that you're taking for another medical condition may cause or contribute to urinary incontinence in a variety of ways, including increasing urine production, obstructing the flow of urine, preventing release of urine (urinary retention), or relaxing of bladder and sphincter muscles.

Be sure to tell your medical provider about all of the medications you take. Your provider may be able to suggest a different dose or medication, or a change in the time you take the medication.

Medications associated with urinary incontinence
- Alpha-adrenergic agonists and alpha-adrenergic antagonists
- Antiarrhythmics
- Anticholinergics and antispasmodics
- Antihistamines and decongestants
- Antiparkinsonian medications
- Antipsychotics
- Benzodiazepines
- Calcium channel blockers
- Diuretics
- Muscle relaxants
- Nonsteroidal anti-inflammatory drugs
- Opioids
- Sedatives
- Serotonin and noradrenaline reuptake inhibitors

Sources: National Institutes of Diabetes and Digestive and Kidney Diseases; Campbell-Walsh-Wein Urology. 12th ed., Elsevier, 2021; Brockle-hurst's Textbook of Geriatric Medicine and Gerontology. 8th ed., Elsevier, 2017; Emergency Medicine Clinic of North America, 2019;37:649.

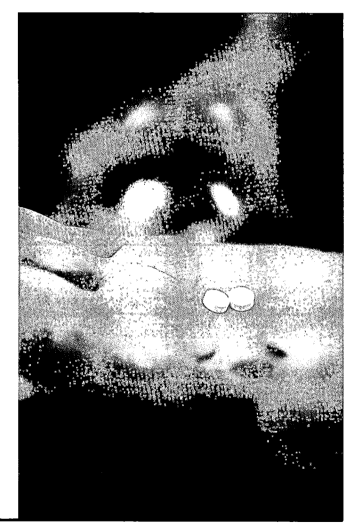

PELVIC FLOOR EXERCISES

Pelvic floor exercises, also called Kegel exercises, involve squeezing and relaxing the muscles in your pelvic and genital area. The exercises help maintain the strength, endurance and proper action of your pelvic floor muscles, which are important for bladder and bowel control. When performed correctly and regularly, pelvic floor exercises can help improve and maintain bladder and bowel control.

How to do the exercises

First, you need to locate your pelvic floor muscles (see page 180). Imagine that you're trying to avoid passing gas in public. The muscles that you use to do that are your pelvic floor muscles. Squeeze and lift the rectal area and, if you're female, the vaginal area, without tightening your buttocks or belly. You should sense a pulling or drawing in feeling in your genital area when you squeeze. Men should try to pull in their penis while also squeezing the anus.

There are three ways to do the exercises:

Endurance contractions

Get into a comfortable position. Strongly tighten — lift and squeeze — your pelvic floor muscles and try to hold the contraction for a count of five (five seconds). At first you may not be able to keep the muscles tightened for very long. If you're not able to hold the contraction for five seconds, then try to hold it for a count of three (three seconds) and gradually increase the time. Rest for 10 seconds between each contraction. Perform 10 repetitions at least three times a day, and practice the exercises in different positions, including while sitting and standing.

Quick flicks

Here, you rapidly contract and release your pelvic floor muscles. Quickly tighten them and hold for one to two seconds. Release the contraction and relax for two seconds. Repeat. Perform 10 repetitions at least three times a day. Again, practice the exercises in different positions.

Urge control

This exercise can be done when you feel a strong urge to urinate or when you're trying to wait longer to go the bathroom. First, stop and stand very still. Sit down if you can. Contract your pelvic muscles quickly and strongly, like the quick flick exercise, five to 10 times. These contractions will signal the bladder that it's not time to empty. Try to think of something other than going to the bathroom. Contract your muscles again if you need to. When you feel the urge lessen somewhat, walk normally to the bathroom. If the urge happens again on the way, stop and repeat the exercise.

Note: Another technique to help reduce urgency is to perform heel raises. Point your toes and then flex your feet, lifting your heels off the ground as high as you can. Do this 10 to 20 times.

You can do pelvic floor muscle exercises almost anywhere — while you're driving, watching TV or sitting at your desk. Ask your doctor how many exercises to do each day. A simple starting program is to do 10 before getting out of bed in the morning, 10 after lunch, 10 in the evening and another 10 before falling asleep.

To see improvements, it's important that you perform at least three sets of 10 repetitions daily. Additional repetitions may produce even better results. After six to 12 weeks of doing pelvic floor exercises correctly, you should notice improvement in your bladder and bowel control.

One way to be sure you're doing the exercises correctly is to place a clean finger in your anus or vagina (for women).

You can do this while you're in the shower or with the help of a rubber glove and a lubricant. Then squeeze around your finger. The muscles you contract are your pelvic floor muscles. If you don't feel anything tighten around your finger, you may need to work with a pelvic floor physical therapist.

To further strengthen the urinary and pelvic floor muscles, some women use vaginal weights. They are tampon-shaped cones that you insert into your vagina and try to hold in place. If you're doing the contractions correctly, you should be able to hold the cone in place. If you aren't doing them correctly, the cone falls out. As your contraction technique improves and your muscles grow stronger, you increase the weight of the cone.

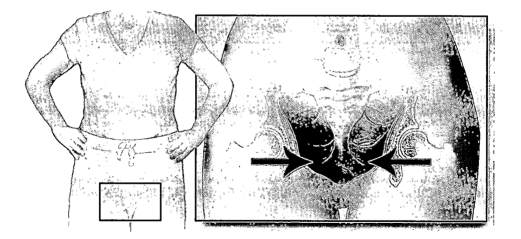

Squeezing pelvic floor muscles that are important to bladder and bowel control will help strengthen the muscles.

BLADDER DRILLS

Bladder drills also are sometimes referred to as timed-voiding exercises. They're a form of bladder training in which you urinate on schedule.

The goal of bladder drills is to improve your ability to remain dry by gradually doing the following:
• Increasing the length of time between your trips to the bathroom
• Increasing the amount of fluid your bladder can hold
• Decreasing the sense of urgency and leakage you experience

Bladder drills generally take place over a period of 12 days or so. It's best to start on a weekend or a day when you plan to be home or near a bathroom. You may want to talk to your doctor before starting this plan.

When following this program, consider these tips:
• Make sure to drink enough fluid every day. Drinking appropriate amounts and emptying your bladder at regular intervals helps decrease the risk of bladder infections.
• Keep a bladder diary (see page 174) as a way to track your progress.

You're the best judge of how quickly you should advance to the next step. The guidelines in the bladder drill schedule below are general suggestions.

BLADDER DRILL SCHEDULE

Days 1 to 3
After waking up, empty your bladder every hour on the hour, even if you don't feel the need to go. Make sure you're drinking at least eight glasses of fluid each day. During the night, only go to the bathroom if you wake up and have to go.

Days 4 to 6
Increase the time between emptying your bladder to every 1½ hours, with the same fluid and night instructions as above.

Days 7 to 9
Increase the time between emptying your bladder to every two hours, with the same fluid and night instructions as above.

Days 10 to 12
Increase the time between emptying your bladder to every 2½ hours, with the same fluid and night instructions as above. Work up to urinating every 3 to 3½ hours.

If the schedule on the previous page doesn't work for you, consider a different pace that works better.

For example, you might decide to change your voiding schedule every two days instead of every three days. Or you may find it more comfortable to increase the time between urinations by 15-minute intervals instead of 30-minute intervals. During days four to six, for example, instead of waiting 1½ hours between trips to the bathroom, wait 1 hour and 15 minutes.

If you feel a sense of urgency to go to the bathroom before your next scheduled time, try doing pelvic floor muscle exercises (see page 179). If possible, sit down until the sensation passes. Remind yourself that your bladder isn't really full, and try to think about something else.

Over several weeks or months, you may find that you can wait up to 3½ hours between trips to the bathroom. Hopefully, you will also find that you have fewer feelings of urgency and fewer episodes of incontinence.

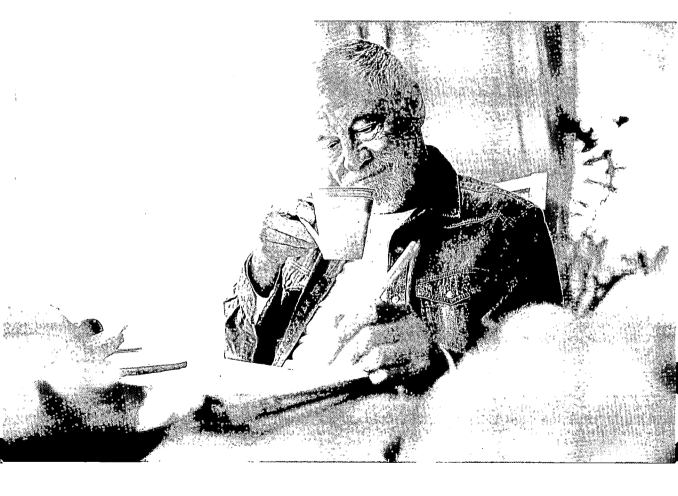

BOWEL DIARY

A bowel diary is often used in conjunction with a food diary — a record of what and when you eat and drink. Together, the two diaries can help determine the cause of fecal incontinence.

Your medical provider will supply you with a diary in which you record the date and time of your bowel movements, the consistency of the stool, whether you felt the urge to empty your bowels, and any episodes of incontinence. It's also helpful to note feelings of straining, discomfort or incomplete emptying. In addition, if you use enemas or laxatives, make note of that.

Doctors generally recommend keeping a bowel diary for at least one week. Choose a time that best represents your normal life. It's best not to keep a diary during vacations or when there are other changes or disruptions in your normal routine.

You can use the bowel diary on pages 184-185 to keep a record of episodes of fecal incontinence. You may want to make copies of the diary and keep them in the bathroom to make it easier to record each episode.

Keeping a bowel diary can be an important first step in determining the cause of your incontinence. A broad range of conditions and disorders can lead to fecal incontinence. To treat the problem, it's imperative to know the cause. By recording episodes of incontinence and important information related to the events, your doctor may be able to determine what may be triggering the episodes.

DIETARY RESTRICTIONS

Some of the things that you eat or drink may irritate your bowels and aggravate fecal incontinence. By keeping a diary of what you eat and drink and your signs and symptoms, you may begin to see a connection between certain foods and beverages and your symptoms.

You can use the diary on page 177 or develop your own. List what you eat and drink, how much, and indicate if you had an episode of incontinence.

After you identify a food or beverage that seems to cause problems, try reducing or eliminating that item from your diet for a week or two. If your signs and symptoms improve, consider avoiding the item permanently or at least reducing how much you consume.

Bowel irritants

Foods and beverages that can cause diarrhea and worsen fecal incontinence include:
- Caffeine
- Cured or smoked meats, such as sausage, ham and turkey
- Spicy foods
- Alcohol
- Dairy products
- Fruits such as apples, peaches and pears
- Fatty and greasy foods
- Sweeteners such as sorbitol, xylitol, mannitol and fructose, which are found in diet drinks, sugarless gum and candy, chocolate, and fruit juices

SAMPLE BOWEL DIARY

Record one bowel episode per column of the diary, even if there is more than one a day. Choose the best answer for each question. Copy the diary as needed.

	Day 1	Day 2	Day 3
Date:			
Time:	a.m. p.m.	a.m. p.m.	a.m. p.m.
Amount of stool:	☐ None ☐ Minor soiling ☐ Staining ☐ Major soiling	☐ None ☐ Minor soiling ☐ Staining ☐ Major soiling	☐ None ☐ Minor soiling ☐ Staining ☐ Major soiling
Do you have to hurry to the toilet?	☐ Yes ☐ No	☐ Yes ☐ No	☐ Yes ☐ No
How long did you hold your bowel movement (minutes):			
Stool description (Circle the number that best describes consistency)*	1 2 3 4 5 6 7	1 2 3 4 5 6 7	1 2 3 4 5 6 7
Did the episode occur while you were sleeping, or did it wake you from sleep?	☐ While sleeping ☐ Woke me	☐ While sleeping ☐ Woke me	☐ While sleeping ☐ Woke me

*Stool consistency: pellets = 1, formed and hard = 2, formed and soft = 3, semiformed = 4, mushy = 5, loose = 6, watery = 7

Day 4	Day 5	Day 6	Day 7
a.m. p.m.	a.m. p.m.	a.m. p.m.	a.m. p.m.
☐ None ☐ Minor soiling ☐ Staining ☐ Major soiling	☐ None ☐ Minor soiling ☐ Staining ☐ Major soiling	☐ None ☐ Minor soiling ☐ Staining ☐ Major soiling	☐ None ☐ Minor soiling ☐ Staining ☐ Major soiling
☐ Yes ☐ No	☐ Yes ☐ No	☐ Yes ☐ No	☐ Yes ☐ No
1 2 3 4 5 6 7	1 2 3 4 5 6 7	1 2 3 4 5 6 7	1 2 3 4 5 6 7
☐ While sleeping ☐ Woke me	☐ While sleeping ☐ Woke me	☐ While sleeping ☐ Woke me	☐ While sleeping ☐ Woke me

PROBLEM MEDICATIONS

Medications that you're taking for another medical condition may cause or contribute to fecal incontinence in a variety of ways, including increased water absorption in the large intestine, disruption of bacteria in the large intestine, a change in muscle tone, and slowed or speedy passage of waste through the digestive tract.

Be sure to tell your doctor or other health care provider about all of the medications you take. Your provider may be able to suggest a different dose or medication, or a change in the time you take the medication.

Medications associated with fecal incontinence
- ACE inhibitors
- Alpha blockers
- Antacids
- Antibiotics
- Anticholinergics
- Anticonvulsants
- Antidepressants and mood stabilizers
- Antifungals
- Antipsychotics
- Antivirals
- Beta blockers
- Bile acid sequestrants
- Chemotherapy drugs
- Diabetic medications
- Laxatives
- Muscle relaxants
- Prostaglandins
- Proton pump inhibitors
- Stimulants

Sources: Obstetrics & Gynecology, 2019;133:e260; Sleisenger and Fordtran's Gastrointestinal and Liver Disease: Pathophysiology, Diagnosis, Management, 11th ed., Elsevier, 2021; Facts & Comparisons eAnswers; UpToDate.

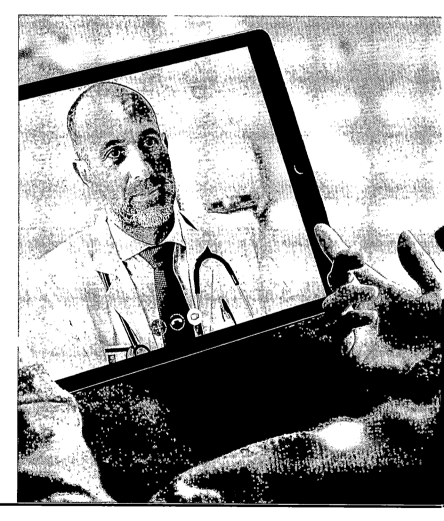

QUESTIONS FOR YOUR DOCTOR

To find a doctor to help with incontinence — urinary or fecal — don't be afraid to ask questions. One of the most important things a doctor can do is to acknowledge your problem with sympathy and support.

Following are some possible questions to think about when choosing a doctor:
- What is the doctor's education and training regarding incontinence? (See page 8 for information on incontinence specialists.)
- How long will you have to wait for an appointment?
- Is the doctor part of your health insurance plan?
- Does the doctor seem concerned about your incontinence and does he or she answer your questions and explain things clearly?
- Does he or she seem knowledgeable about incontinence treatments?

Once you've chosen a medical provider, you may have questions about diagnostic tests, medications or treatment.

About tests
- What will this test show?
- How accurate is it?
- Are there any risks or side effects?
- Will it be uncomfortable?
- Do I need to do anything special before or after the test?

About medications
- Why do I need this medication?
- Are there any side effects?
- When should my symptoms improve?
- Are there any special instructions?

About treatments
- What are the benefits and risks?
- When can I expect to see improvement in my condition?
- Are there other treatments available?
- Can you refer me to another doctor for a second opinion?
- If surgery is needed, how long will I be hospitalized?
- What's the average recovery time?
- Can my condition be cured?
- What incontinence and skin care products would help me manage better?

Additional resources

Alliance for Aging Research
202-293-2856 • www.agingresearch.org

American Urogynecologic Society
301-273-0570 • www.augs.org

Health in Aging
212-308-1414 • www.healthinaging.org

International Continence Society
www.ics.org

International Foundation for
Gastrointestinal Disorders
414-964-1799 • www.iffgd.org

National Association For Continence
800-252-3337 • www.nafc.org

National Digestive Diseases
Information Clearinghouse
800-860-8747 • niddk.nih.gov

National Institute on Aging
800-222-2225 • www.nia.nih.gov

National Institutes of Health
301-496-4000 • www.nih.gov

National Kidney and Urologic Diseases
Information Clearinghouse
800-860-8747 • niddk.nih.gov

Office on Women's Health
800-994-9662 • www.womenshealth.gov

The Simon Foundation for Continence
800-237-4666 • www.simonfoundation.org

Urology Care Foundation
800-828-7866 • www.urologyhealth.org

Index

K

Kegels
  See pelvic floor exercises
key-in-the-hole syndrome, 18
kidneys
  about, 14
  aging and, 28
  congestive heart failure and, 34
  diabetes and, 35
  illustrated, 13
  overflow incontinence and, 20

L

laxatives, 164
leak point pressure measurement, 50
leakage, urine, 120
lifestyle changes (urinary incontinence)
  fluid and diet management, 55-57
  medications, changing, 57-58
  physical activity, increasing, 59
  smoking cessation, 59
  weight management, 58-59
living well with incontinence
  environment modification and, 117
  getting out and, 117-119
  risk reduction and, 113-117
loperamide (Imodium A-D), 164
lower urinary tract, 14-16
lubiprostone (Amitiza), 164

M

magnetic resonance imaging (MRI), 53,
    150-151
male exam, urinary incontinence, 46-47
manometry, 146-147, 162
meal portions and timing, 158
medical history
  fecal incontinence and, 142-144
  urinary incontinence and, 39-40, 42

medications
  changing, as lifestyle change, 57-58
  constipation, 164
  diarrhea, 164
  for fecal incontinence, 163-164
  as fecal incontinence cause, 136, 144,
    159
  problem (fecal incontinence), 186
  problem (urinary incontinence), 178
  as urinary incontinence cause, 20, 25,
    43, 57-58
medications (urinary incontinence)
  about, 53, 71-72
  alpha-adrenergic blockers, 74
  anticholinergics, 72-74
  antidepressants, 78-79
  beta-3 adrenergic agonists, 74
  desmopressin, 79
  effective but too dangerous, 75
  estrogen, topical, 75-77
  table of, 76-77
men
  bladder control issues and, 13
  compression products, 65
  overflow incontinence in, 19-20
  physical examination (urinary
    incontinence), 46-47
  sexuality and incontinence and, 120-121
  stress incontinence in, 17
  urethra, 14-15
  urge incontinence in, 18
  urinary incontinence in, 98-102
  urinary tract, 13
menopause and urinary incontinence,
    12-13, 29-30, 96
methylphenidate (Ritalin), 107
mixed incontinence, 18-19, 58
mobility, restricted, 34
multiple sclerosis, urinary incontinence
    and, 18, 35-36
muscle damage, fecal incontinence and,
    134

MAYO CLINIC

Reliable resources from the hospital ranked #1 in the nation

From disease management to healthy living, you and your family can trust the expert guidance from Mayo Clinic.

Learn more today by visiting
Marketplace.MayoClinic.com

U.S. News & World Report, 2020-2021

MAYO CLINIC | mayoclinic.org

©2021 Mayo Foundation for Medical Education and Research. All rights reserved. MAYO, MAYO CLINIC and the triple-shield Mayo logo are trademarks and service marks of MFMER.